PARKINSON'S DIET COOKBOOK FOR BEGINNERS

A Flavorful 21-Day Culinary Adventure for Optimal Well-being"

George F. Quint

Copyright © 2024

All Rights Are Reserved

The content in this book may not be reproduced, duplicated, or transferred without the express written permission of the author or publisher. Under no circumstances will the publisher or author be held liable or legally responsible for any losses, expenditures, or damages incurred directly or indirectly as a consequence of the information included in this book.

Legal Remarks

Copyright protection applies to this publication. It is only intended for personal use. No piece of this work may be modified, distributed, sold, quoted, or paraphrased without the author's or publisher's consent.

Disclaimer Statement

Please keep in mind that the contents of this booklet are meant for educational and recreational purposes. Every effort has been made to offer accurate, up-to-date, reliable, and thorough information. There are, however, no stated or implied assurances of any kind. Readers understand that the author is providing competent counsel. The content in this book originates from several sources. Please seek the opinion of a competent professional before using any of the tactics outlined in this book. By reading this book, the reader agrees that the author will not be held accountable for any direct or indirect damages resulting from the use of the information contained therein, including, but not limited to, errors, omissions, or inaccuracies.

TABLE OF CONTENTS

CHAPTER TWELVE...252

EXERCISE AND NUTRITION SYNERGY.................252

CHAPTER THIRTHEEN.......................................263

EMOTIONAL WELL-BEING AND NUTRITION......263

CONCLUSION..273

INTRODUCTION

Understanding Parkinson's Disease

Parkinson's Disease (PD) is a complex neurodegenerative disorder that significantly impacts the lives of those diagnosed and their families. From a neurological perspective, PD is characterized by the gradual degeneration of dopamine-producing neurons in the brain, particularly in the substantia nigari. This depletion of dopamine, a neurotransmitter critical for smooth, controlled movement, leads to the hallmark motor symptoms associated with Parkinson's.

The clinical manifestation of Parkinson's is diverse, encompassing both motor and non-motor symptoms. Motor symptoms include tremors, bradykinesia (slowness of movement), rigidity, and postural instability, while non-motor symptoms range from cognitive impairment and mood disorders to autonomic dysfunction. The variability and progression of these symptoms contribute to the complexity of managing the condition.

Understanding the multifaceted nature of Parkinson's Disease requires an exploration of its origins. While genetic factors play a role, environmental triggers, such as exposure to certain toxins, are also implicated.

Advancing age is a significant risk factor, and there are subtle gender distinctions in prevalence and symptomatology. A definitive diagnosis involves a thorough clinical evaluation, often supplemented by neuroimaging and other diagnostic tests to differentiate PD from other neurodegenerative conditions.

Currently, treatment strategies for Parkinson's Disease primarily focus on managing symptoms. Medications, including dopamine agonists and levodopa, are commonly prescribed. In more advanced cases, surgical interventions like deep brain stimulation may be considered. Complementary non-pharmacological approaches, such as physical therapy and occupational therapy, are integral components of comprehensive care.

Living with Parkinson's presents unique challenges, both for individuals affected and their support networks. Coping strategies, adaptive technologies, and a strong support system become essential elements in enhancing the quality of life for those navigating this journey. Moreover, dispelling myths and addressing stigmas associated with Parkinson's is crucial in fostering understanding and empathy within communities.

The landscape of Parkinson's research is dynamic and promising. Ongoing studies explore novel therapeutic avenues, from neuroprotective agents to gene therapies, offering hope for improved treatment modalities and, ultimately, a cure. Acknowledging the prevalent misconceptions about Parkinson's is vital in fostering awareness and advocacy, contributing to a more informed and supportive global community.

Importance of Diet in Managing Parkinson's Symptoms

Parkinson's Disease (PD) is not only a neurological challenge but also a condition where the role of diet becomes increasingly apparent in managing symptoms and promoting overall well-being. This chapter delves into the critical connection between nutrition and Parkinson's, emphasizing the impact dietary choices can have on symptom management and quality of life.

Nutritional Foundations for Parkinson's Patients

- ***Holistic Approach:*** Understanding nutrition as an integral part of a holistic approach to Parkinson's management.

- ***Nutrient Requirements:*** Exploring the specific nutrient needs of individuals with Parkinson's and how these may differ from the general population.

Diet's Influence on Neurotransmitters

- ***Dopamine Support:*** Identifying dietary elements that support dopamine production and availability in the brain.

- ***Balancing Neurotransmitters:*** Examining the interplay between various neurotransmitters affected by diet and their impact on motor and non-motor symptoms.

Inflammation and Antioxidants

- ***Inflammation Connection:*** Understanding the link between inflammation and Parkinson's symptoms.

- ***Antioxidant-Rich Foods:*** Exploring the role of antioxidants in mitigating oxidative stress and inflammation, with a focus on specific foods.

Gut-Brain Axis and Dietary Impact

- ***Gut Health Significance:*** Investigating the emerging research on the gut-brain axis and its relevance to Parkinson's.

- ***Probiotics and Prebiotics:*** Considering the potential benefits of incorporating these elements into the diet for gut health.

Managing Medication Efficacy through Diet

- ***Interaction Awareness:*** Recognizing how certain foods may interact with Parkinson's medications.

- ***Optimizing Medication Absorption:*** Strategies for ensuring optimal absorption of medications through dietary choices.

Hydration as a Fundamental Element

- ***Fluid Intake Guidelines:*** Discussing the importance of proper hydration in managing symptoms and potential medication side effects.

- ***Hydration Challenges:*** Addressing common hydration challenges faced by Parkinson's patients and offering practical solutions.

Personalized Dietary Approaches

- ***Individual Variability:*** Acknowledging the diverse nutritional needs and preferences of individuals with Parkinson's.

- ***Tailoring Diets:*** Exploring approaches to tailor diets to suit the unique requirements and sensitivities of each patient.

Collaborating with Healthcare Professionals

- ***Dietitian's Role:*** Understanding the contribution of dietitians and healthcare professionals in crafting personalized dietary plans.

- ***Interdisciplinary Care:*** Emphasizing the importance of collaboration between neurologists, dietitians, and other healthcare providers.

Real-World Application: Success Stories

- ***Patient Testimonials:*** Showcasing real-life success stories where dietary changes positively impacted Parkinson's symptoms.

- ***Practical Tips:*** Offering practical tips and strategies for incorporating a Parkinson's-friendly diet into daily life.

Long-Term Benefits and Considerations

- ***Quality of Life Improvement:*** Highlighting the potential long-term benefits of maintaining a healthy and Parkinson's-appropriate diet.

- ***Sustainability:*** Discussing strategies for making dietary changes sustainable and enjoyable over the course of Parkinson's progression.

CHAPTER ONE

FOUNDATIONS OF A PARKINSON'S-FRIENDLY DIET

Overview of a Nutrient-Rich Diet

In the pursuit of managing Parkinson's Disease effectively, a cornerstone lies in the implementation of a nutrient-rich diet. This section provides a comprehensive exploration of the key elements that constitute a nutrient-rich diet, emphasizing the vital role these components play in supporting overall health for individuals living with Parkinson's.

Defining Nutrient-Rich Diets

- *Holistic Nutrition:* Understanding the concept of nutrient richness as a holistic approach to nourishing the body.

- *Beyond Calories:* Shifting the focus from calorie quantity to nutrient quality for optimal well-being.

Essential Macronutrients for Parkinson's Patients

- *Balancing Carbohydrates:* Exploring the significance of complex carbohydrates in providing sustained energy levels.

- *Protein Considerations:* Discussing the role of protein intake in supporting muscle function while managing potential medication interactions.

- *Healthy Fats:* Recognizing the importance of incorporating sources of healthy fats for brain health and overall balance.

Micronutrients: The Building Blocks of Health

- *Vitamins and Minerals:* Detailing the critical role of various vitamins and minerals in promoting cellular function and overall health.

- *Antioxidants:* Emphasizing the importance of antioxidants in mitigating oxidative stress and inflammation.

The Power of Whole Foods

- *Whole Foods vs. Processed Foods:* Understanding the nutritional superiority of whole, unprocessed foods.

- *Incorporating Variety:* Encouraging a diverse and colorful array of fruits, vegetables, and whole grains for maximum nutritional benefit.

Hydration as a Fundamental Component

- *Importance of Hydration:* Underscoring the role of proper hydration in supporting bodily functions and medication efficacy.

- *Hydrating Foods:* Identifying foods with high water content that contribute to overall fluid intake.

Tailoring Nutrient-Rich Diets to Parkinson's Needs

- *Individualized Approaches:* Recognizing the unique nutritional needs and sensitivities of individuals living with Parkinson's.

- *Dietary Modifications:* Discussing potential adjustments based on medication interactions and symptom management.

Dietary Challenges and Solutions

- *Addressing Dietary Challenges:* Acknowledging common obstacles individuals with Parkinson's may face in maintaining a nutrient-rich diet.

- *Practical Solutions:* Offering practical tips and strategies to overcome these challenges and foster dietary adherence.

Collaborating with Nutrition Professionals

- *Role of Dietitians:* Highlighting the significance of partnering with registered dietitians for personalized nutritional guidance.

- *Interdisciplinary Care:* Emphasizing collaboration between healthcare professionals to optimize dietary support for Parkinson's patients.

Key Nutrients for Parkinson's Patients

To effectively navigate the challenges posed by Parkinson's Disease, a nuanced understanding of essential nutrients becomes paramount. This section delves into the specific nutrients crucial for individuals with Parkinson's, shedding light on their roles in symptom management, overall well-being, and potential interactions with medications.

Vitamin D: The Sunshine Nutrient

- **Bone Health:** Examining the role of vitamin D in maintaining bone density, especially relevant for Parkinson's patients at risk of falls.

- **Potential Neuroprotective Effects:** Discussing emerging research on the connection between vitamin D and neuroprotection.

Omega-3 Fatty Acids: Brain Boosters

- ***Brain Health Benefits:*** Unpacking the role of omega-3 fatty acids, particularly EPA and DHA, in supporting cognitive function.

- ***Inflammation Modulation:*** Exploring how omega-3s may contribute to managing inflammation, a factor in Parkinson's progression.

Antioxidants: Cellular Defenders

- ***Combatting Oxidative Stress:*** Understanding how antioxidants, including vitamins C and E, can help counteract oxidative stress associated with Parkinson's.

- ***Polyphenols and Flavonoids:*** Exploring the potential benefits of these plant compounds in promoting brain health.

B Vitamins: Energy and Neurotransmitter Support

- ***Role in Energy Metabolism:*** Discussing how B vitamins, including B6, B9 (folate), and B12, contribute to energy production.

- ***Neurotransmitter Synthesis:*** Highlighting their role in the synthesis of neurotransmitters, crucial for managing Parkinson's symptoms.

Magnesium: Muscle and Nerve Function

- ***Muscle Relaxation:*** Understanding how magnesium can help alleviate muscle stiffness and cramping common in Parkinson's.

- ***Neurological Stability:*** Exploring the potential impact of magnesium on nerve function and overall neurological stability.

Coenzyme Q10: Mitochondrial Support

- ***Mitochondrial Function:*** Investigating the role of CoQ10 in supporting mitochondrial function, potentially beneficial for energy production.

- ***Neuroprotective Effects:*** Examining the antioxidant and neuroprotective properties of CoQ10 in the context of Parkinson's.

Iron: Balance and Regulation

- ***Iron Levels in Parkinson's:*** Addressing the delicate balance of iron levels and potential considerations for Parkinson's patients.

- ***Impact on Medication Absorption:*** Discussing how iron intake may influence the absorption of Parkinson's medications.

Protein: Moderation and Medication Optimization

- ***Balancing Protein Intake:*** Navigating the delicate balance of protein intake for muscle health while considering potential interactions with medication.

- ***Timing and Distribution:*** Discussing strategies for optimizing protein consumption throughout the day for enhanced medication efficacy.

Fiber: Gut Health and Constipation Management

- ***Gut-Brain Connection:*** Understanding the role of fiber in supporting gut health and its potential impact on neurological well-being.

- ***Constipation Management:*** Exploring how adequate fiber intake can help alleviate a common symptom of Parkinson's.

The Role of Hydration

In the comprehensive approach to managing Parkinson's Disease, the significance of hydration emerges as a critical aspect influencing both physical well-being and medication efficacy. This section explores the multifaceted role of hydration and offers insights into optimizing fluid intake for individuals living with Parkinson's.

Understanding Hydration in Parkinson's

- ***Fluid Balance:*** Examining the importance of maintaining proper fluid balance in individuals with Parkinson's to support bodily functions.

- ***Potential Impact on Symptoms:*** Exploring how hydration levels can influence common symptoms such as fatigue, muscle cramps, and cognitive function.

Medication Absorption and Hydration

- ***Hydration and Medication Efficacy:*** Investigating the connection between hydration status and the absorption of Parkinson's medications.

- ***Optimizing Medication Administration:*** Offering practical tips for coordinating medication schedules with hydration routines.

Hydration Challenges in Parkinson's

- ***Swallowing Difficulties:*** Addressing the challenges individuals with Parkinson's may face due to swallowing difficulties and their impact on fluid intake.

- ***Timing and Frequency:*** Discussing strategies to overcome challenges related to timing and frequency of fluid intake throughout the day.

Hydrating Foods and Beverages

- ***Water-Rich Foods:*** Identifying foods with high water content as an additional source of hydration.

- ***Balancing Beverages:*** Offering a variety of beverage options that contribute to hydration while considering factors such as caffeine and sugar content.

Dehydration Risk Factors and Prevention

- ***Environmental Factors:*** Recognizing how environmental factors, such as temperature and humidity, may contribute to dehydration risk.

- ***Individual Susceptibility:*** Discussing factors that may increase susceptibility to dehydration and strategies for prevention.

Monitoring Hydration Levels

- ***Visual and Physical Indicators:*** Providing guidance on recognizing signs of dehydration through physical cues, such as urine color and skin condition.

- ***Technological Solutions:*** Exploring the use of technology, such as hydration apps and smart water bottles, to facilitate regular monitoring.

Hydration and Physical Activity

- ***Exercise Considerations:*** Addressing the impact of hydration on physical activity and providing guidelines for maintaining fluid balance during exercise.

- ***Rehydration Post-Exercise:*** Offering recommendations for effective rehydration following physical activity.

Collaborating with Healthcare Professionals

- ***Role of Healthcare Providers:*** Emphasizing the importance of communication with healthcare professionals, including neurologists and dietitians, to address hydration concerns.

- ***Individualized Hydration Plans:*** Discussing the development of personalized hydration plans tailored to the unique needs of individuals with Parkinson's.

CHAPTER TWO

BUILDING A BALANCED PLATE

Portion Control and Meal Frequency

In the realm of Parkinson's management, establishing optimal portion sizes and meal frequency plays a pivotal role in maintaining energy levels, managing symptoms, and supporting overall well-being. This chapter delves into the significance of portion control and meal frequency for individuals living with Parkinson's, offering practical guidance for navigating these dietary aspects effectively.

Importance of Portion Control

- ***Energy Balance:*** Exploring the concept of energy balance and the role of portion control in managing calorie intake.

- ***Symptom Management:*** Discussing how appropriate portion sizes can help alleviate symptoms such as digestive discomfort and fluctuations in energy levels.

Tailoring Portion Sizes to Individual Needs

- ***Personalized Approach:*** Recognizing the importance of individual variability in determining optimal portion sizes based on factors such as age, weight, and activity level.

* **Medication Considerations:** Addressing how Parkinson's medications may influence appetite and metabolism, impacting portion size requirements.

Strategies for Portion Control

* **Plate Method:** Introducing the plate method as a practical tool for visualizing portion sizes and balancing macronutrients.

* **Using Portion-Controlled Servings:** Discussing the benefits of pre-portioned meals and snacks for promoting portion control and convenience.

Understanding Meal Frequency

* **Balancing Frequency and Volume:** Exploring the relationship between meal frequency and portion sizes in optimizing energy distribution throughout the day.

* **Effects on Blood Sugar Levels:** Discussing how regular meal intervals can help stabilize blood sugar levels and prevent energy crashes.

Practical Tips for Meal Frequency

- ***Consistent Timing:*** Recommending regular meal and snack times to establish a predictable eating routine and maintain metabolic balance.

- ***Balanced Snacking:*** Providing suggestions for nutrient-dense snacks that can be incorporated between meals to support energy levels and manage hunger.

Adapting Meal Frequency to Lifestyle and Symptoms

- ***Flexibility and Adaptability:*** Encouraging individuals to adjust meal frequency based on lifestyle factors, appetite cues, and symptom fluctuations.

- ***Symptom Management Strategies:*** Offering guidance on modifying meal frequency to address specific symptoms such as dysphagia or medication-related side effects.

Hydration and Meal Timing

- ***Hydration Integration:*** Discussing the importance of coordinating fluid intake with meals and snacks to support hydration and digestion.

- ***Hydration Between Meals:*** Emphasizing the need for adequate hydration between meals to maintain fluid balance and prevent dehydration.

Monitoring and Adjusting

- ***Self-Awareness:*** Encouraging individuals to tune into hunger and fullness cues to guide portion sizes and meal frequency adjustments.

- ***Tracking and Evaluation:*** Recommending the use of food journals or apps to monitor eating patterns and assess the effectiveness of portion control and meal frequency strategies.

Collaborating with Healthcare Professionals

- ***Role of Dietitians:*** Highlighting the importance of consulting with registered dietitians to develop personalized portion control and meal frequency plans.

- ***Interdisciplinary Care:*** Emphasizing collaboration between healthcare professionals to address nutritional needs comprehensively within the context of Parkinson's management.

Creating Balanced Meals for Energy and Sustenance

In the realm of Parkinson's Disease management, crafting well-balanced meals is a fundamental component, crucial for sustaining energy levels, managing symptoms, and promoting overall health. This section explores the principles of designing meals that cater specifically to the unique needs of individuals living with Parkinson's.

The Plate Method for Parkinson's Patients

- ***Visualizing a Balanced Plate:*** Introducing the plate method as an effective tool for designing nutritionally balanced meals.

- ***Adapting to Individual Needs:*** Discussing how the plate method can be tailored to accommodate individual dietary preferences, restrictions, and nutritional requirements.

Prioritizing Nutrient-Rich Foods

- ***Incorporating Parkinson's Superfoods:*** Identifying nutrient-dense foods, including antioxidants, omega-3 fatty acids, and vitamins crucial for Parkinson's management.

- ***Balancing Macronutrients:*** Ensuring an appropriate distribution of carbohydrates, proteins, and healthy fats for sustained energy.

Timing and Frequency of Meals

- ***Optimizing Meal Timing:*** Discussing the importance of meal timing in relation to medication schedules and symptom management.

- ***Considerations for Snacking:*** Exploring the role of nutritious snacks in maintaining consistent energy levels throughout the day.

Hydration as a Meal Component

- ***Incorporating Hydrating Foods:*** Highlighting the significance of integrating water-rich foods into meals for both nutrition and hydration.

- ***Timing of Hydration:*** Discussing considerations for fluid intake during meals and its potential impact on digestion.

Addressing Swallowing Difficulties

- ***Texture-Modified Diets:*** Exploring strategies for adapting meal textures to accommodate individuals with swallowing difficulties.

- ***Nutrient Density in Soft Diets:*** Ensuring nutritional adequacy in softer-textured meals.

Cooking Techniques for Parkinson's Patients

- ***Simplified Cooking Methods:*** Offering practical cooking techniques that streamline meal preparation for individuals with motor challenges.

- ***Batch Cooking and Meal Prepping:*** Discussing the benefits of batch cooking and meal prepping for convenience and consistency.

Cultural and Personal Preferences

- *Respecting Individual Preferences:* Emphasizing the importance of incorporating cultural and personal food preferences into meal planning.

- *Exploring Global Cuisine:* Showcasing diverse and Parkinson's-friendly recipes from various culinary traditions.

Collaborating with Nutrition Professionals

- ***Consulting with Dietitians:*** Stressing the value of collaboration with registered dietitians in tailoring meal plans to individual needs.

- ***Adapting Meal Plans Over Time:*** Discussing the dynamic nature of dietary adjustments, especially as Parkinson's symptoms evolve.

The Plate Method for Parkinson's Patients

In the pursuit of optimal nutrition for Parkinson's patients, the Plate Method emerges as a valuable and practical tool for creating balanced meals. This section explores the principles and applications of the Plate Method, tailoring its implementation to the unique needs and considerations of individuals living with Parkinson's.

Understanding the Plate Method

- ***Visual Representation:*** Introducing the Plate Method as a visual guide that divides the plate into specific sections for different food groups.

- ***Balancing Macronutrients:*** Emphasizing the importance of incorporating a balance of carbohydrates, proteins, and healthy fats for sustained energy.

Adapting the Plate Method for Parkinson's

- ***Individualized Approach:*** Recognizing the need for customization based on individual dietary preferences, restrictions, and Parkinson's-related challenges.

- ***Medication Timing Considerations:*** Discussing how the Plate Method can be aligned with medication schedules to optimize energy levels and symptom management.

Filling the Plate with Nutrient-Rich Foods

- ***Prioritizing Superfoods:*** Incorporating Parkinson's superfoods rich in antioxidants, omega-3 fatty acids, and vitamins.

- ***Emphasizing Color and Variety:*** Encouraging a diverse array of colorful fruits, vegetables, and whole grains to maximize nutritional benefits.

Hydration Integration

- ***Incorporating Hydrating Foods:*** Highlighting the role of water-rich foods within the Plate Method to address hydration needs.

- ***Balancing Fluid Intake:*** Discussing considerations for fluid intake alongside meals to support overall hydration.

Practical Tips for Plate Method Success

- ***Portion Control:*** Emphasizing the importance of appropriate portion sizes within each section of the plate.

- ***Mindful Eating:*** Introducing mindful eating practices, such as savoring each bite and paying attention to hunger and fullness cues.

Meal Timing and Frequency

- ***Aligning with Medication Schedule:*** Discussing strategies for meal timing to complement Parkinson's medication schedules.

- ***Snacking Considerations:*** Exploring the role of nutritious snacks in maintaining energy levels between meals.

Addressing Swallowing Difficulties with the Plate Method

- ***Texture Modifications:*** Adapting the Plate Method to accommodate individuals with swallowing difficulties through texture modifications.

- ***Ensuring Nutrient Density:*** Ensuring that softer-textured meals maintain nutritional adequacy.

Culinary Creativity with the Plate Method

- ***Simplified Cooking Techniques:*** Incorporating cooking techniques that align with motor challenges, ensuring accessibility and ease.

- ***Global Cuisine Exploration:*** Encouraging the exploration of diverse Parkinson's-friendly recipes from various cultural traditions.

Progression and Adaptation

- ***Dynamic Nature:*** Acknowledging the dynamic nature of Parkinson's symptoms and the need for ongoing adaptation of the Plate Method.

- ***Collaboration with Dietitians****:* Highlighting the collaborative role of registered dietitians in tailoring and adjusting the Plate Method over time.

CHAPTER THREE

PARKINSON'S SUPERFOODS

In the realm of Parkinson's Disease management, incorporating nutrient-dense foods, commonly referred to as "superfoods," holds tremendous potential for supporting overall health and potentially mitigating certain symptoms. This chapter introduces the concept of superfoods, delving into their nutritional significance and exploring how they can be integrated into the diet of individuals living with Parkinson's.

Defining Superfoods in the Context of Parkinson's

- ***Nutrient Density:*** Understanding the term "superfood" in relation to foods that are rich in essential nutrients, antioxidants, and other bioactive compounds.

- ***Potential Benefits for Parkinson's Patients:*** Discussing how the unique nutritional profiles of superfoods may contribute to symptom management and overall well-being.

Antioxidant-Rich Superfoods for Neuroprotection

- ***Role of Antioxidants:*** Exploring the significance of antioxidants in combating oxidative stress, a factor associated with Parkinson's progression.

- ***Berries:*** Highlighting the neuroprotective properties of berries, rich in anthocyanins and other antioxidants.

Omega-3 Fatty Acid Sources for Brain Health

- ***Importance of Omega-3s:*** Discussing the role of omega-3 fatty acids in supporting brain health and potentially alleviating cognitive symptoms.

- ***Fatty Fish:*** Identifying fatty fish, such as salmon and mackerel, as valuable sources of omega-3s.

Leafy Greens and their Nutritional Power

- ***Rich in Vitamins and Minerals:*** Exploring how leafy greens provide essential vitamins and minerals crucial for overall health.

- ***Kale, Spinach, and Swiss Chard:*** Showcasing specific leafy greens and their nutritional contributions.

Nuts and Seeds as Nutrient Powerhouses

- ***Healthy Fats and Protein:*** Discussing the benefits of nuts and seeds, which offer a combination of healthy fats, protein, and essential nutrients.

- ***Walnuts, Flaxseeds, and Chia Seeds:*** Examining the nutritional profiles of specific nuts and seeds.

Colorful Fruits and Vegetables for a Vibrant Diet

- ***Phytochemical Diversity:*** Emphasizing the importance of consuming a variety of colorful fruits and vegetables for a diverse array of phytochemicals.

- ***Oranges, Bell Peppers, and Sweet Potatoes:*** Showcasing vibrant produce and their nutritional contributions.

Incorporating Superfoods into Everyday Meals

- ***Smoothies and Bowls:*** Offering creative and practical ways to incorporate superfoods into daily meals, such as through smoothies and bowls.

- ***Recipe Ideas:*** Providing simple and delicious recipes that feature superfoods and cater to the specific dietary needs of individuals with Parkinson's.

Potential Considerations and Interactions

- ***Consulting Healthcare Professionals:*** Emphasizing the importance of consulting with healthcare professionals, particularly dietitians, to ensure that superfoods align with individual health needs and potential medication interactions.

- ***Balancing Superfoods in the Diet:*** Discussing the need for balance and moderation in incorporating superfoods to maintain a well-rounded and sustainable diet.

Incorporating Antioxidant-Rich Foods

In the quest for optimal health and Parkinson's management, the integration of antioxidant-rich foods stands out as a strategic dietary approach. This section explores the significance of antioxidants, their potential benefits in managing oxidative stress associated with Parkinson's, and practical strategies for seamlessly incorporating these foods into the daily diet.

Understanding the Role of Antioxidants in Parkinson's Management

- ***Mitigating Oxidative Stress:*** Examining how oxidative stress is implicated in Parkinson's progression and the protective role of antioxidants.

- ***Neuroprotection:*** Discussing the potential neuroprotective effects of antioxidants in supporting overall brain health.

Key Antioxidant Nutrients for Parkinson's Patients

- ***Vitamin C:*** Exploring the role of vitamin C in neutralizing free radicals and its sources in fruits and vegetables.

- ***Vitamin E:*** Discussing the antioxidant properties of vitamin E and its presence in nuts, seeds, and leafy greens.

Berries: A Potent Source of Antioxidants

- ***Anthocyanins and Flavonoids:*** Highlighting the antioxidant-rich compounds, such as anthocyanins, present in berries.

- ***Incorporating Berries into the Diet:*** Offering creative ways to include berries in meals, snacks, and desserts.

Dark Leafy Greens and their Antioxidant Content

- ***Rich in Vitamins A and C:*** Discussing how dark leafy greens contribute to antioxidant intake through vitamins A and C.

- ***Kale and Spinach Recipes:*** Providing recipes that showcase dark leafy greens in appetizing and nutrient-rich dishes.

Nuts and Seeds: Antioxidant-Packed Snacking Options

- ***Selenium and Zinc Content:*** Exploring how nuts and seeds, rich in selenium and zinc, contribute to antioxidant defense.

- ***Nut and Seed Mixes:*** Suggesting flavorful combinations for creating antioxidant-packed snack mixes.

Colorful Fruits and Vegetables for a Diverse Antioxidant Palette

- ***Phytochemical Diversity:*** Emphasizing the importance of consuming a spectrum of colorful fruits and vegetables for a diverse range of antioxidants.

- ***Rainbow Salad Ideas:*** Inspiring the creation of visually appealing salads incorporating a variety of colorful produce.

Herbal Teas and Spices with Antioxidant Properties

- ***Polyphenol-Rich Teas:*** Introducing herbal teas with high polyphenol content and their potential antioxidant benefits.

- ***Spices for Flavor and Health:*** Exploring how spices like turmeric and cinnamon can contribute to antioxidant intake.

Practical Tips for Antioxidant-Rich Meal Planning

- ***Weekly Meal Prep Strategies:*** Offering practical guidance on incorporating antioxidant-rich foods into weekly meal planning.

- ***Seasonal Eating:*** Advocating for the inclusion of seasonal fruits and vegetables to maximize antioxidant diversity.

Monitoring and Adjusting Antioxidant Intake

- ***Tracking Dietary Patterns:*** Discussing the potential benefits of keeping a food diary to monitor antioxidant intake.

- ***Adapting to Changing Needs:*** Recognizing the importance of adjusting antioxidant intake based on individual health status and progression of Parkinson's.

Omega-3 Fatty Acids for Brain Health

In the pursuit of holistic well-being for individuals managing Parkinson's Disease, the focus on omega-3 fatty acids emerges as a key dietary consideration. This chapter explores the critical role of omega-3s in supporting brain health, managing cognitive function, and potentially mitigating certain symptoms associated with Parkinson's.

The Significance of Omega-3 Fatty Acids in Neurological Health

- **Essential Fatty Acids:** Introducing omega-3 fatty acids as essential components crucial for brain structure and function.

- **DHA and EPA:** Highlighting the specific importance of docosahexaenoic acid (DHA) and eicosapentaenoic acid (EPA) in neurological well-being.

Cognitive Benefits of Omega-3s in Parkinson's

- **Cognitive Support:** Examining the potential role of omega-3s in supporting cognitive function, memory, and concentration.

- **Reducing Cognitive Decline:** Discussing research on the correlation between omega-3 intake and a potential reduction in cognitive decline.

Fatty Fish as Rich Sources of Omega-3s

- ***Salmon, Mackerel, and Trout:*** Identifying specific fatty fish rich in omega-3s and their potential inclusion in a Parkinson's-friendly diet.

- ***Incorporating Fatty Fish into Meals:*** Offering creative and accessible recipes that feature omega-3-rich fish.

Plant-Based Sources of Omega-3s for Non-Fish Eaters

- ***Chia Seeds and Flaxseeds:*** Exploring plant-based alternatives for individuals who do not consume fish.

- ***Omega-3 Enriched Foods:*** Discussing fortified foods as additional sources of omega-3s for plant-based diets.

Anti-Inflammatory Effects of Omega-3s in Parkinson's

- ***Managing Inflammation:*** Investigating the potential anti-inflammatory effects of omega-3s and their relevance to Parkinson's symptoms.

- ***Balancing Omega-6 and Omega-3 Ratios:*** Discussing the importance of maintaining a balanced ratio of omega-6 to omega-3 fatty acids.

Supplements and Omega-3 Intake

- ***Consulting with Healthcare Professionals:*** Emphasizing the need for consultation with healthcare providers, particularly neurologists and dietitians, before incorporating omega-3 supplements.

- ***Choosing High-Quality Supplements:*** Providing guidance on selecting reputable and well-formulated omega-3 supplements.

Practical Tips for Including Omega-3s in Daily Meals

- ***Meal Planning Strategies:*** Offering practical tips for incorporating omega-3-rich foods into daily meal planning.

- ***Diverse Omega-3 Sources:*** Encouraging a diverse selection of omega-3 sources to maximize nutritional benefits.

Monitoring and Adjusting Omega-3 Intake

- ***Tracking Dietary Patterns:*** Discussing the potential benefits of keeping a food diary to monitor omega-3 intake.

- ***Adapting to Individual Needs:*** Recognizing the importance of adjusting omega-3 intake based on individual health status and progression of Parkinson's.

CHAPTER FOUR

FOODS TO LIMIT OR AVOID

Understanding Trigger Foods

Navigating the dietary landscape in Parkinson's Disease management requires a nuanced awareness of trigger foods - those that may exacerbate symptoms or interfere with medication effectiveness. This chapter explores the concept of trigger foods, identifies common culprits, and provides guidance on recognizing and managing their impact.

Defining Trigger Foods in the Context of Parkinson's

- ***Impact on Symptoms:*** Understanding trigger foods as those that may worsen specific Parkinson's symptoms.

- ***Individual Variability:*** Acknowledging that trigger foods can vary among individuals, and their effects may be influenced by factors such as medication regimens and overall health.

Common Culprits: Foods to Approach with Caution

- ***High-Protein Foods:*** Recognizing the potential interference of high-protein foods with levodopa absorption and their impact on medication effectiveness.

- **Caffeine and Its Effects:** Discussing how caffeine may affect sleep patterns, exacerbate tremors, or interact with medications.

Assessing Personal Sensitivities

- **Keeping a Food Diary:** Encouraging individuals with Parkinson's to maintain a food diary to identify patterns between diet and symptom exacerbation.

- **Consulting Healthcare Professionals:** Stressing the importance of involving healthcare providers, particularly dietitians, in assessing personal sensitivities.

Trigger Foods and Gastrointestinal Symptoms

- **Constipation Triggers:** Identifying foods that may contribute to constipation, a common symptom in Parkinson's.

- **Addressing Digestive Discomfort:** Offering dietary strategies to manage gastrointestinal symptoms and improve digestive comfort.

Sodium and Fluid Intake Considerations

- ***Fluid Retention and Medications:*** Discussing the potential impact of high sodium intake on fluid retention, which may influence medication efficacy.

- ***Balancing Hydration:*** Emphasizing the importance of maintaining adequate hydration while being mindful of sodium levels.

Managing Nutrient Interactions with Medications

- ***Timing of Medication and Meals:*** Advising on the importance of timing meals to minimize potential nutrient interactions with Parkinson's medications.

- ***Individualized Medication Plans:*** Highlighting the need for personalized strategies, as the impact of trigger foods may vary based on individual medication regimens.

Lifestyle Factors and Trigger Food Sensitivity

- ***Stress and Emotional Eating:*** Addressing how stress and emotional factors may influence sensitivity to trigger foods.

- ***Lifestyle Modifications:*** Discussing lifestyle changes, such as regular exercise and stress management, that can complement dietary adjustments.

Developing Personalized Dietary Plans

- *Collaboration with Dietitians:* Emphasizing the crucial role of registered dietitians in crafting personalized dietary plans.

- *Trial and Error Approaches:* Recognizing that identifying trigger foods often involves a process of trial and error, requiring patience and diligence.

Managing Medication Interactions

Effectively managing Parkinson's Disease involves not only dietary considerations but also a keen awareness of potential interactions between medications and various substances. This chapter delves into the nuances of medication interactions, offering guidance on optimizing medication effectiveness, minimizing side effects, and fostering a comprehensive approach to Parkinson's management.

Understanding Parkinson's Medications

- *Levodopa and Dopamine Agonists:* Providing an overview of common medications used in

Parkinson's treatment and their mechanisms of action.

- ***Complementary Medications:*** Discussing additional medications prescribed to address specific symptoms or enhance the effects of primary medications.

The Impact of Diet on Medication Absorption

- ***High-Protein Interactions:*** Exploring how dietary protein can influence the absorption of levodopa, a key medication in Parkinson's treatment.

- ***Optimizing Medication Timing:*** Advising on strategic meal planning and protein intake timing to minimize interference with medication absorption.

Nutritional Considerations for Medication Efficacy

- ***Balancing Nutrient Intake:*** Discussing the importance of maintaining a well-balanced diet to ensure adequate nutrients for overall health and support medication effectiveness.

- ***Vitamin and Mineral Supplements:*** Advising on the cautious use of supplements, considering potential interactions with medications.

5.4 Caffeine and its Impact on Medications

- ***Caffeine and Dopamine Production:*** Discussing the potential effects of caffeine on dopamine production and its implications for individuals taking dopamine-related medications.

- ***Balancing Caffeine Intake:*** Providing recommendations on moderate caffeine consumption to minimize potential interference with medications.

Sodium Levels and Medication Interactions

- ***Fluid Retention and Blood Pressure Medications:*** Addressing the impact of high sodium intake on fluid retention and potential interactions with medications targeting blood pressure.

- ***Balancing Sodium Intake:*** Providing guidelines on maintaining a balanced sodium intake to support both cardiovascular health and medication efficacy.

Alcohol and its Effects on Parkinson's Medications

- ***Central Nervous System Depressant Effects:*** Exploring how alcohol, as a central nervous system depressant, may interact with medications affecting the nervous system.

- ***Moderation and Monitoring:*** Advising on the importance of moderate alcohol consumption and vigilant monitoring of any adverse effects.

Collaboration with Healthcare Professionals

- ***Communication with Neurologists and Dietitians:*** Emphasizing the significance of open communication with healthcare professionals, particularly neurologists and dietitians, regarding dietary habits and potential interactions.

- ***Periodic Medication Reviews:*** Discussing the importance of regular reviews of medications and potential adjustments based on individual responses.

Lifestyle Factors and Medication Management

- ***Exercise and Medication Effects:*** Recognizing the potential influence of exercise on medication absorption and effectiveness.

- ***Stress Management:*** Discussing the role of stress in Parkinson's symptoms and strategies for stress reduction, which may positively impact medication responses.

Caffeine, Alcohol, and Other Considerations

In the multifaceted landscape of Parkinson's management, specific substances such as caffeine and alcohol warrant careful consideration due to their potential impact on symptoms and medication efficacy. This chapter explores the nuanced effects of caffeine, alcohol, and other factors, providing guidance on incorporating them judiciously into the daily lives of individuals living with Parkinson's.

Caffeine and Parkinson's Symptoms

- ***Cognitive Effects:*** Discussing the potential cognitive benefits and challenges associated with caffeine consumption in individuals with Parkinson's.

- ***Motor Symptoms:*** Exploring the impact of caffeine on motor symptoms, including tremors and muscle stiffness.

Strategic Caffeine Consumption

- ***Timing and Quantity:*** Advising on the optimal timing and moderate quantities of caffeine intake to harness potential benefits while minimizing negative effects.

- ***Personal Sensitivity:*** Recognizing individual variations in caffeine sensitivity and its potential influence on symptom responses.

Alcohol and its Effects on Parkinson's Symptoms

- ***Motor Function and Balance:*** Discussing how alcohol consumption may affect motor function and balance, factors crucial for individuals with Parkinson's.

- ***Interactions with Medications:*** Addressing potential interactions between alcohol and Parkinson's medications, emphasizing the need for moderation.

Moderation and Personalized Approaches

- ***Individual Responses:*** Recognizing the importance of individualized approaches to caffeine and alcohol consumption based on personal sensitivities and responses.

- ***Consulting Healthcare Professionals:*** Emphasizing the role of healthcare professionals, including neurologists and dietitians, in guiding personalized approaches.

Tobacco and Parkinson's Risk

- ***Nicotine and Dopamine Release:*** Discussing the potential link between nicotine, found in tobacco, and increased dopamine release, which may influence Parkinson's risk.

- ***Balancing Risks and Benefits:*** Encouraging individuals to weigh the potential risks of tobacco use against its possible impact on Parkinson's development.

Environmental Factors and Parkinson's Risk

- ***Pesticide Exposure:*** Discussing the association between pesticide exposure and an increased risk of Parkinson's.

- ***Protective Measures:*** Advising on precautions, such as using protective gear during gardening, to minimize exposure to environmental toxins.

Stress Management for Parkinson's Patients

- ***Impact on Symptoms:*** Exploring the connection between stress and the exacerbation of Parkinson's symptoms.

- ***Mind-Body Techniques:*** Introducing stress management techniques, including mindfulness and relaxation exercises, to alleviate psychological stress.

Incorporating Social and Recreational Activities

- ***Community Engagement:*** Emphasizing the importance of social interactions and recreational activities in promoting mental well-being for individuals with Parkinson's.

- ***Balancing Activities:*** Advising on finding a balance between social engagement and the need for rest and self-care.

Emotional Well-being and Parkinson's

- ***Depression and Anxiety:*** Addressing the prevalence of depression and anxiety in individuals with Parkinson's and the importance of seeking professional support.

- ***Holistic Approaches:*** Promoting a holistic approach to emotional well-being, encompassing social support, therapy, and self-care practices.

CHAPTER FIVE

BREAKFAST RECIPES

Nutrient-Packed Smoothie Bowl

Ingredients:

- 1 cup mixed berries (strawberries, blueberries, raspberries)

- 1 ripe banana

- 1/2 cup spinach leaves

- 1 tablespoon chia seeds

- 1/2 cup low-fat Greek yogurt

- 1/2 cup almond milk

Preparation Time: 10 minutes

Cooking Time: 0 minutes

Serving Time: 5 minutes

Nutritional Info: High in antioxidants, fiber, and essential vitamins.

Instructions:

- Blend berries, banana, spinach, chia seeds, Greek yogurt, and almond milk until smooth.

- Pour into a bowl.

- Top with sliced fruits, nuts, and a drizzle of honey.

Serving Methods:

1. As a refreshing breakfast bowl.

2. Freeze into popsicle molds for a tasty and cooling treat.

Quinoa and Vegetable Breakfast Skillet

Ingredients:

- 1 cup cooked quinoa

- 1/2 cup bell peppers (red and green), diced

- 1/4 cup red onion, finely chopped

- 1/2 cup cherry tomatoes, halved

- 2 eggs

- 1 tablespoon olive oil

- Salt and pepper to taste

Preparation Time: *15 minutes*

Cooking Time: *15 minutes*

Serving Time: *5 minutes*

Nutritional Info: *High in protein, fiber, and essential nutrients*

Instructions:

- In a skillet, sauté onions and bell peppers in olive oil until softened.

- Add cherry tomatoes and cooked quinoa, stirring well.

- Create small wells in the mixture and crack eggs into them.

- Cover and cook until eggs are set.

- Season with salt and pepper.

Serving Methods:

1. Serve as a hearty skillet meal.

2. Spoon onto whole-grain toast for a breakfast bruschetta.

Oatmeal with Almond Butter and Berries

Ingredients:

- 1/2 cup rolled oats

- 1 cup water or milk of choice

- 1 tablespoon almond butter

- 1/2 cup mixed berries (strawberries, blackberries)

- 1 teaspoon honey (optional)

- 1 tablespoon chopped almonds

Preparation Time: 5 minutes

Cooking Time: 10 minutes

Serving Time: 5 minutes

Nutritional Info: Rich in fiber, healthy fats, and antioxidants.

Instructions:

- Cook oats with water or milk according to package instructions.

- Stir in almond butter until well combined.

- Top with mixed berries, honey, and chopped almonds.

Serving Methods:

1. Enjoy as a warm bowl of oatmeal.

2. Freeze leftovers in molds for an oatmeal popsicle.

Sweet Potato and Spinach Frittata

Ingredients:

- 1 medium sweet potato, grated

- 1 cup fresh spinach leaves, chopped

- 4 eggs

- 1/4 cup milk

- 1/4 cup feta cheese, crumbled

- Salt and pepper to taste

- 1 tablespoon olive oil

Preparation Time: 15 minutes

Cooking Time: 20 minutes

Serving Time: 5 minutes

Nutritional Info: High in vitamins, minerals, and protein.

Instructions:

- Preheat oven to 350°F (175°C).

- In an oven-safe skillet, sauté sweet potato in olive oil until softened.

- Add spinach and cook until wilted.

- Whisk eggs with milk, salt, and pepper. Pour over vegetables.

- Sprinkle feta cheese on top and bake until eggs are set.

Serving Methods:

1. Serve wedges warm from the skillet.

2. Chill and slice into squares for a grab-and-go breakfast.

Chia Seed Pudding with Mango

Ingredients:

- 3 tablespoons chia seeds
- 1 cup almond milk
- 1/2 teaspoon vanilla extract
- 1 tablespoon honey
- 1 ripe mango, diced
- 1 tablespoon shredded coconut

Preparation Time: 5 minutes

Cooking Time: 0 minutes

Serving Time: 2 hours (for pudding to set)

Nutritional Info: Packed with omega-3s, fiber, and natural sweetness.

Instructions:

- Mix chia seeds, almond milk, vanilla extract, and honey in a jar.

- Refrigerate for at least 2 hours or overnight until a pudding consistency is achieved.

- Top with diced mango and shredded coconut.

Serving Methods:

1. Spoon into a bowl for a traditional pudding experience.

2. Layer with granola and yogurt for a parfait.

Avocado and Smoked Salmon Toast

Ingredients:

- 1 slice whole-grain bread

- 1/2 ripe avocado, mashed

- 50g smoked salmon

- 1 tablespoon capers

- Fresh dill for garnish

- Lemon wedges

Preparation Time: 10 minutes

Cooking Time: 0 minutes

Serving Time: 5 minutes

Nutritional Info: Rich in omega-3s, fiber, and healthy fats.

Instructions:

- Toast the whole-grain bread to your liking.

- Spread mashed avocado on the toast.

- Top with smoked salmon, capers, and fresh dill.

- Serve with lemon wedges for extra flavor.

Serving Methods:

1. Enjoy as an open-faced sandwich.

2. Cut into bite-sized pieces for a savory appetizer.

Coconut Yogurt Parfait with Berries

Ingredients:

- 1 cup coconut yogurt

- 1/2 cup granola (low sugar)

- 1/2 cup mixed berries (blueberries, raspberries)

- 1 tablespoon honey

- 1 tablespoon shredded coconut

Preparation Time: 5 minutes

Cooking Time: 0 minutes

Serving Time: 5 minutes

Nutritional Info: High in probiotics, antioxidants, and fiber.

Instructions:

- In a glass, layer coconut yogurt, granola, and mixed berries.

- Drizzle honey over the layers.

- Top with shredded coconut.

Serving Methods:

1. Serve in a tall glass for an elegant presentation.

2. Mix all ingredients together for a quick and easy breakfast bowl.

Spinach and Mushroom Egg Muffins

Ingredients:

- 4 eggs

- 1 cup fresh spinach, chopped

- 1/2 cup mushrooms, diced

- 1/4 cup feta cheese, crumbled

- Salt and pepper to taste

- Cooking spray

Preparation Time: 10 minutes

Cooking Time: 20 minutes

Serving Time: 5 minutes

Nutritional Info: High in protein, vitamins, and minerals.

Instructions:

- Preheat the oven to 375°F (190°C) and grease a muffin tin with cooking spray.

- In a bowl, whisk eggs and season with salt and pepper.

- Stir in chopped spinach, mushrooms, and feta cheese.

- Pour the mixture into the muffin tin and bake until set.

Serving Methods:

1. Serve warm as a protein-packed breakfast.

2. Refrigerate leftovers and enjoy cold for a quick snack.

Blueberry Almond Pancakes

Ingredients:

- 1 cup almond flour

- 2 eggs

- 1/2 cup almond milk

- 1/2 teaspoon baking powder

- 1/2 cup blueberries (fresh or frozen)

- Maple syrup for drizzling

Preparation Time: 15 minutes

Cooking Time: 10 minutes

Serving Time: 5 minutes

Nutritional Info: Gluten-free, high in protein, and antioxidants.

Instructions:

- In a bowl, whisk almond flour, eggs, almond milk, and baking powder until smooth.

- Gently fold in blueberries.

- Spoon batter onto a hot griddle and cook until golden brown on both sides.

- Drizzle with maple syrup before serving.

Serving Methods:

1. Stack pancakes on a plate for a classic presentation.

2. Cut into smaller pieces and serve as finger foods for convenience.

Mango and Banana Breakfast Wrap

Ingredients:

- 1 whole-grain tortilla

- 1/2 cup Greek yogurt

- 1 ripe banana, sliced

- 1/2 ripe mango, diced

- 1 tablespoon chia seeds

- Drizzle of honey

Preparation Time: 10 minutes

Cooking Time: 0 minutes

Serving Time: 5 minutes

Nutritional Info: High in fiber, vitamins, and probiotics.

Instructions:

- Spread Greek yogurt on the whole-grain tortilla.

- Arrange banana slices and diced mango on top.

- Sprinkle chia seeds and drizzle with honey.

- Fold the tortilla into a wrap and secure with a toothpick if needed.

Serving Methods:

1. Slice the wrap into bite-sized pinwheels for a delightful brunch.

2. Serve as a whole wrap with a side of fresh berries for a balanced meal.

Quinoa Breakfast Bowl

Ingredients:

- 1/2 cup cooked quinoa

- 1/4 cup sliced almonds

- 1/2 cup mixed berries (strawberries, blueberries)

- 1 tablespoon honey

- 1/2 cup low-fat Greek yogurt

- 1 teaspoon chia seeds

Preparation Time: 10 minutes

Cooking Time: 15 minutes

Serving Time: 5 minutes

Nutritional Info: High in protein, fiber, and antioxidants.

Instructions:

- Combine quinoa, sliced almonds, and mixed berries in a bowl.

- Drizzle with honey and top with Greek yogurt.

- Sprinkle chia seeds over the top.

Serving Methods:

1. Serve in a breakfast bowl.

2. Layer ingredients in a mason jar for a portable option.

Sweet Potato and Turkey Sausage Hash

Ingredients:

- 1 medium sweet potato, diced

- 1/2 cup lean turkey sausage, crumbled

- 1/4 cup red bell pepper, chopped

- 1/4 cup onion, diced

- 2 eggs

- 1 tablespoon olive oil

- Salt and pepper to taste

Preparation Time: 15 minutes

Cooking Time: 20 minutes

Serving Time: 5 minutes

Nutritional Info: Rich in vitamins, protein, and healthy fats.

Instructions:

- In a skillet, sauté sweet potato, turkey sausage, bell pepper, and onion in olive oil until cooked.

- Create wells in the mixture and crack eggs into them.

- Cover and cook until eggs are set.

- Season with salt and pepper.

Serving Methods:

1. Serve in a bowl with a poached egg on top.

2. Wrap the hash in a whole-grain tortilla for a breakfast burrito.

Almond Butter Banana Muffins

Ingredients:

- 2 ripe bananas, mashed

- 1/2 cup almond butter

- 2 eggs

- 1 teaspoon vanilla extract

- 1 cup almond flour

- 1/2 teaspoon baking soda

- 1/4 teaspoon salt

Preparation Time: 15 minutes

Cooking Time: 20 minutes

Serving Time: 5 minutes

Nutritional Info: Gluten-free, high in protein, and healthy fats.

Instructions:

- Preheat the oven to 350°F (175°C) and line a muffin tin.

- In a bowl, mix mashed bananas, almond butter, eggs, and vanilla extract.

- Add almond flour, baking soda, and salt. Mix until combined.

- Spoon batter into muffin cups and bake until a toothpick comes out clean.

Serving Methods:

1. Enjoy muffins warm with a dollop of Greek yogurt.

2. Slice and spread with cream cheese for a savory twist.

Mushroom and Spinach Omelette

Ingredients:

- 3 eggs

- 1/2 cup mushrooms, sliced

- 1 cup fresh spinach

- 1/4 cup feta cheese, crumbled

- 1 tablespoon olive oil

- Salt and pepper to taste

Preparation Time: 10 minutes

Cooking Time: 10 minutes

Serving Time: 5 minutes

Nutritional Info: High in protein, vitamins, and minerals

Instructions:

- In a skillet, sauté mushrooms and spinach in olive oil until wilted.

- Whisk eggs in a bowl and pour over the vegetables.

- Sprinkle feta cheese on one half of the omelette.

- Fold the omelette in half and cook until eggs are set.

Serving Methods:

1. Serve the omelette on a plate with a side of sliced avocado.

2. Roll the omelette and slice into pinwheels for a visually appealing option.

Pumpkin Spice Chia Pudding

Ingredients:

- 3 tablespoons chia seeds

- 1 cup unsweetened almond milk

- 1/4 cup pumpkin puree

- 1/2 teaspoon pumpkin spice

- 1 tablespoon maple syrup

- 1/4 cup chopped walnuts

Preparation Time: 5 minutes

Cooking Time: 0 minutes

Serving Time: 2 hours (for pudding to set)

Nutritional Info: Rich in omega-3s, fiber, and autumn flavors.

Instructions:

- Mix chia seeds, almond milk, pumpkin puree, pumpkin spice, and maple syrup in a jar.

- Refrigerate for at least 2 hours or overnight until a pudding consistency is achieved.

- Top with chopped walnuts before serving.

Serving Methods:

1. Spoon into a bowl for a traditional pudding experience.

2. Layer with granola and yogurt for a parfait.

Cauliflower and Broccoli Breakfast Bake

Ingredients:

- 1 cup cauliflower florets, steamed

- 1 cup broccoli florets, steamed

- 4 eggs

- 1/2 cup shredded cheddar cheese

- 1/4 cup diced red bell pepper

- Salt and pepper to taste

Preparation Time: 15 minutes

Cooking Time: 25 minutes

Serving Time: 5 minutes

Nutritional Info: High in fiber, protein, and essential nutrients.

Instructions:

- Preheat the oven to 375°F (190°C) and grease a baking dish.

- Layer cauliflower and broccoli in the dish.

- Whisk eggs, add diced red bell pepper, and season with salt and pepper.

- Pour the egg mixture over the vegetables and top with shredded cheddar cheese.

- Bake until eggs are set and the top is golden brown.

Serving Methods:

1. Cut into squares for a breakfast casserole.

2. Serve alongside a side of mixed greens for a complete meal.

Turmeric and Ginger Golden Milk Smoothie

Ingredients:

- 1 cup unsweetened coconut milk

- 1/2 teaspoon ground turmeric

- 1/2 teaspoon ground ginger

- 1 banana

- 1 tablespoon almond butter

- 1/2 teaspoon honey

- Ice cubes

Preparation Time: 5 minutes

Cooking Time: 0 minutes

Serving Time: 5 minutes

Nutritional Info: Anti-inflammatory, rich in antioxidants, and energy-boosting

Instructions:

- Blend coconut milk, turmeric, ginger, banana, almond butter, and honey until smooth.

- Add ice cubes and blend again until desired consistency.

Serving *Methods*:

1. Pour into a glass for a refreshing smoothie.

2. Freeze into popsicle molds for a cool treat.

Green Pea and Mint Frittata

***Ingredients*:**

- 4 eggs

- 1/2 cup green peas (fresh or frozen)

- 2 tablespoons fresh mint, chopped

- 1/4 cup goat cheese, crumbled

- 1 tablespoon olive oil

- Salt and pepper to taste

Preparation Time: 10 minutes

Cooking Time: 15 minutes

Serving Time: 5 minutes

Nutritional Info: High in protein, vitamins, and refreshing flavors.

Instructions:

- Preheat the oven to 350°F (175°C).

- In a skillet, sauté green peas in olive oil until tender.

- Whisk eggs, add mint, goat cheese, salt, and pepper.

- Pour the egg mixture over the peas and transfer to the oven.

- Bake until the frittata is set and golden brown.

Serving Methods:

1. Serve wedges warm with a side of mixed greens.

2. Allow to cool and cut into bite-sized squares for a party appetizer.

Apple Cinnamon Breakfast Quinoa

Ingredients:

- 1/2 cup cooked quinoa

- 1 apple, diced

- 1/4 cup chopped walnuts

- 1/2 teaspoon cinnamon

- 1 tablespoon maple syrup

- 1/2 cup vanilla-flavored Greek yogurt

Preparation Time: 10 minutes

Cooking Time: 15 minutes

Serving Time: 5 minutes

Nutritional Info: High in fiber, antioxidants, and protein.

Instructions:

- Mix cooked quinoa, diced apple, chopped walnuts, cinnamon, and maple syrup in a bowl.

- Serve with a dollop of vanilla-flavored Greek yogurt on top.

Serving Methods:

1. Enjoy in a breakfast bowl for a hearty start.

2. Layer ingredients in a glass for a visually appealing parfait.

Lemon Poppy Seed Pancakes

Ingredients:

- 1 cup whole wheat flour

- 1 tablespoon poppy seeds

- 1 teaspoon baking powder

- 1/2 teaspoon baking soda

- 1/4 teaspoon salt

- 1 cup buttermilk

- 1 egg

- Zest of 1 lemon

- 1 tablespoon lemon juice

- 1 tablespoon honey

Preparation Time: 15 minutes

Cooking Time: 10 minutes

Serving Time: 5 minutes

Nutritional Info: High in fiber, vitamin C, and a delightful citrus flavor.

Instructions:

- In a bowl, whisk together flour, poppy seeds, baking powder, baking soda, and salt.

- In another bowl, whisk buttermilk, egg, lemon zest, lemon juice, and honey.

- Combine wet and dry ingredients until just mixed.

- Cook pancakes on a griddle until golden brown on both sides.

Serving Methods:

1. Stack pancakes on a plate with a drizzle of honey.

2. Roll pancakes with a layer of Greek yogurt for a grab-and-go option.

CHAPTER SIX

LUNCH RECIPES

Salmon and Quinoa Salad

Ingredients:

- 1 cup cooked quinoa

- 150g grilled salmon, flaked

- 1 cup mixed greens (spinach, arugula)

- 1/2 cucumber, sliced

- 1/4 cup cherry tomatoes, halved

- 1 tablespoon olive oil

- 1 tablespoon balsamic vinegar

- Salt and pepper to taste

Preparation Time: 15 minutes

Cooking Time: 15 minutes

Serving Time: 5 minutes

Nutritional Info: Rich in omega-3s, protein, and antioxidants.

Instructions:

- In a bowl, combine quinoa, flaked salmon, mixed greens, cucumber, and cherry tomatoes.

- Whisk together olive oil, balsamic vinegar, salt, and pepper for the dressing.

- Drizzle the dressing over the salad and toss gently.

Serving Methods:

1. Serve in a large bowl for a satisfying lunch.

2. Fill whole-grain wraps with the salad for a portable option.

Turkey and Avocado Lettuce Wraps

Ingredients:

- 200g lean ground turkey

- 1/2 teaspoon cumin

- 1/2 teaspoon paprika

- 1/4 teaspoon garlic powder

- 4 large lettuce leaves

- 1 avocado, sliced

- 1/4 cup salsa

- Fresh cilantro for garnish

Preparation Time: 10 minutes

Cooking Time: 15 minutes

Serving Time: 5 minutes

Nutritional Info: Low-carb, high in protein, and heart-healthy fats.

Instructions:

- In a skillet, cook ground turkey with cumin, paprika, and garlic powder until browned.

- Spoon the turkey mixture onto lettuce leaves.

- Top with avocado slices, salsa, and garnish with fresh cilantro.

Serving Methods:

1. Arrange as an open-faced dish for a light lunch.

2. Roll the lettuce wraps and secure with toothpicks

Vegetarian Quinoa Stuffed Peppers

Ingredients:

- 2 bell peppers, halved and seeds removed

- 1 cup cooked quinoa

- 1/2 cup black beans, drained and rinsed

- 1/2 cup corn kernels

- 1/4 cup diced red onion

- 1/2 cup salsa

- 1/2 teaspoon cumin

- 1/2 teaspoon chili powder

- 1/4 cup shredded cheddar cheese

Preparation Time: 20 minutes

Cooking Time: 25 minutes

Serving Time: 5 minutes

Nutritional Info: High in fiber, plant-based protein, and vitamins.

Instructions:

- Preheat the oven to 375°F (190°C).

- In a bowl, mix quinoa, black beans, corn, red onion, salsa, cumin, and chili powder.

- Stuff the bell peppers with the quinoa mixture.

- Top with shredded cheddar cheese and bake until peppers are tender.

Serving Methods:

1. Serve as a colorful and flavorful main course.

2. Slice into halves for a visually appealing side dish.

Chicken and Broccoli Stir-Fry

Ingredients:

- 200g boneless, skinless chicken breast, sliced

- 1 cup broccoli florets

- 1/2 cup sliced bell peppers (red and yellow)

- 2 tablespoons low-sodium soy sauce

- 1 tablespoon hoisin sauce

- 1 tablespoon sesame oil

- 1 teaspoon ginger, minced

- 1 teaspoon garlic, minced

- Brown rice for serving

Preparation Time: 15 minutes

Cooking Time: 15 minutes

Serving Time: 5 minutes

Nutritional Info: High in protein, fiber, and essential nutrients.

Instructions:

- In a wok or skillet, heat sesame oil and sauté chicken until browned.

- Add broccoli, bell peppers, ginger, and garlic. Stir-fry until vegetables are tender-crisp.

- Pour in soy sauce and hoisin sauce, tossing until everything is coated.

- Serve over brown rice.

Serving Methods:

- Enjoy as a traditional stir-fry with rice.

- Wrap the stir-fry in lettuce leaves for a low-carb option.

Mediterranean Chickpea Salad

Ingredients:

- 1 can (15 oz.) chickpeas, drained and rinsed

- 1 cup cherry tomatoes, halved

- 1/2 cucumber, diced

- 1/4 cup red onion, finely chopped

- 1/4 cup feta cheese, crumbled

- 2 tablespoons Kalamata olives, sliced

- 2 tablespoons extra virgin olive oil

- 1 tablespoon balsamic vinegar

- Fresh oregano for garnish

Preparation Time: 10 minutes

Cooking Time: 0 minutes

Serving Time: 5 minutes

Nutritional Info: High in fiber, plant-based protein, and healthy fats.

Instructions:

- In a large bowl, combine chickpeas, cherry tomatoes, cucumber, red onion, feta cheese, and olives.

- Drizzle with olive oil and balsamic vinegar. Toss gently.

- Garnish with fresh oregano before serving.

Serving Methods:

1. Serve as a refreshing salad.

2. Spoon onto whole-grain pita for a Mediterranean-inspired sandwich.

Tofu and Vegetable Quiche

Ingredients:

- 1 ready-made whole-grain pie crust

- 200g firm tofu, crumbled

- 1 cup mixed vegetables (bell peppers, spinach, mushrooms), chopped

- 1/2 cup cherry tomatoes, halved

- 4 eggs

- 1/2 cup unsweetened almond milk

- 1/4 cup nutritional yeast

- Salt and pepper to taste

Preparation Time: 15 minutes

Cooking Time: 35 minutes

Serving Time: 5 minutes

Nutritional Info: High in plant-based protein, vitamins, and minerals.

Instructions:

- Preheat the oven to 375°F (190°C).

- In a skillet, sauté tofu and mixed vegetables until softened.

- In a bowl, whisk eggs, almond milk, nutritional yeast, salt, and pepper.

- Place the pie crust in a pie dish. Add the tofu-vegetable mixture and cherry tomatoes.

- Pour the egg mixture over the top and bake until set.

Serving Methods:

1. Serve wedges warm for a comforting lunch.

2. Chill and slice into squares for a picnic-friendly option.

Spaghetti Squash with Pesto and Cherry Tomatoes

Ingredients:

- 1 medium spaghetti squash, halved and seeds removed

- 1 cup cherry tomatoes, halved

- 1/4 cup pine nuts, toasted

- 1/2 cup fresh basil leaves

- 1/4 cup Parmesan cheese, grated

- 2 tablespoons olive oil

- Salt and pepper to taste

Preparation Time: 10 minutes

Cooking Time: 45 minutes

Serving Time: 5 minutes

Nutritional Info: Low-carb, rich in vitamins, and healthy fats.

Instructions:

- Preheat the oven to 375°F (190°C).

- Place the spaghetti squash halves on a baking sheet, cut side down.

- Roast until the squash is tender.

- In a blender, combine basil, pine nuts, Parmesan, olive oil, salt, and pepper to make pesto.

- Use a fork to scrape the spaghetti squash into strands. Mix with pesto and cherry tomatoes.

Serving Methods:

1. Serve in the squash halves for an elegant presentation.

2. Spoon into bowls and sprinkle with extra Parmesan for added flavor.

Shrimp and Asparagus Stir-Fry

Ingredients:

- 200g shrimp, peeled and deveined
- 1 bunch asparagus, trimmed and cut into bite-sized pieces
- 1 red bell pepper, sliced
- 2 tablespoons low-sodium soy sauce
- 1 tablespoon rice vinegar
- 1 tablespoon honey
- 1 tablespoon sesame oil
- 1 teaspoon ginger, minced
- 1 teaspoon garlic, minced
- Brown rice for serving

Preparation Time: 15 minutes

Cooking Time: 15 minutes

Serving Time: 5 minutes

Nutritional Info: High in protein, fiber, and essential nutrients.

Instructions:

- In a wok or skillet, heat sesame oil and stir-fry shrimp until pink.

- Add asparagus and bell pepper, continuing to stir-fry until vegetables are tender-crisp.

- In a small bowl, whisk together soy sauce, rice vinegar, honey, ginger, and garlic.

- Pour the sauce over the shrimp and vegetables. Stir until well-coated.

- Serve over brown rice.

Serving Methods:

1. Enjoy as a traditional stir-fry.

2. Spoon the stir-fry into lettuce cups for a light and carb-conscious option.

Cauliflower Rice Burrito Bowl

Ingredients:

- 1 cup cauliflower rice, cooked

- 1/2 cup black beans, drained and rinsed

- 1/2 cup corn kernels

- 1/4 cup diced tomatoes

- 1/4 cup diced red onion

- 1/4 cup shredded lettuce

- 2 tablespoons salsa

- 1 tablespoon Greek yogurt

- Fresh cilantro for garnish

Preparation Time: 10 minutes

Cooking Time: 10 minutes

Serving Time: 5 minutes

Nutritional Info: Low-carb, high in fiber, and plant-based protein.

Instructions:

- In a bowl, layer cauliflower rice, black beans, corn, tomatoes, red onion, and shredded lettuce.

- Drizzle with salsa and Greek yogurt.

- Garnish with fresh cilantro.

Serving Methods:

1. Serve in a bowl for a wholesome lunch.

2. Spoon into bell pepper halves for a creative presentation.

Eggplant and Chickpea Stew

Ingredients:

- 1 large eggplant, diced

- 1 can (15 oz.) chickpeas, drained and rinsed

- 1 cup cherry tomatoes, halved

- 1 onion, diced

- 2 cloves garlic, minced

- 1 teaspoon cumin

- 1 teaspoon paprika

- 1/2 teaspoon cinnamon

- 1 can (14 oz.) crushed tomatoes

- 2 cups vegetable broth

- Fresh parsley for garnish

Preparation Time: 15 minutes

Cooking Time: 30 minutes

Serving Time: 5 minutes

Nutritional Info: High in fiber, plant-based protein, and rich in antioxidants.

Instructions:

- In a large pot, sauté onion and garlic until softened.

- Add diced eggplant, chickpeas, cherry tomatoes, cumin, paprika, and cinnamon. Stir well.

- Pour in crushed tomatoes and vegetable broth. Simmer until eggplant is tender.

- Garnish with fresh parsley before serving.

Serving Methods:

1. Serve in bowls with a slice of whole-grain bread.

2. Spoon over a bed of quinoa for a protein-packed meal.

Salmon and Asparagus Quinoa Bowl

Ingredients:

- 200g salmon fillet

- 1 cup quinoa, cooked

- 1 bunch asparagus, trimmed

- 1 tablespoon olive oil

- 1 lemon, juiced

- Salt and pepper to taste

Preparation Time: 10 minutes

Cooking Time: 15 minutes

Serving Time: 5 minutes

Nutritional Info: High in omega-3s, protein, and fiber.

Instructions:

- Preheat the oven to 400°F (200°C).

- Season salmon with salt, pepper, and a drizzle of olive oil. Bake for 12-15 minutes.

- Sauté asparagus in olive oil until tender.

- Arrange cooked quinoa, asparagus, and salmon in a bowl. Drizzle with lemon juice.

Serving Methods:

1. Serve in a bowl for a wholesome lunch.

2. Wrap ingredients in seaweed for a salmon and quinoa hand roll.

Vegetarian Lentil and Spinach Soup

Ingredients:

- 1 cup dried green lentils

- 1 onion, diced

- 2 carrots, chopped

- 2 celery stalks, sliced

- 3 cups fresh spinach

- 4 cups vegetable broth

- 1 teaspoon cumin

- 1 teaspoon paprika

- Salt and pepper to taste

Preparation Time: 15 minutes

Cooking Time: 30 minutes

Serving Time: 5 minutes

Nutritional Info: High in protein, fiber, and iron.

Instructions:

- Rinse lentils and cook in vegetable broth until tender.

- Sauté onions, carrots, and celery until softened.

- Add cumin, paprika, salt, and pepper.

- Combine sautéed vegetables, lentils, and fresh spinach. Simmer until spinach wilts.

Serving Methods:

1. Ladle into bowls for a comforting soup.

2. Pour over cooked quinoa for a hearty stew.

Chicken and Vegetable Stir-Fry with Brown Rice

Ingredients:

- 200g chicken breast, sliced

- 1 cup broccoli florets

- 1 bell pepper, sliced

- 1 carrot, julienned

- 2 tablespoons low-sodium soy sauce

- 1 tablespoon hoisin sauce

- 1 tablespoon sesame oil

- 1 cup brown rice, cooked

Preparation Time: 15 minutes

Cooking Time: 20 minutes

Serving Time: 5 minutes

Nutritional Info: High in protein, fiber, and essential nutrients.

Instructions:

- Stir-fry chicken in sesame oil until cooked through.

- Add broccoli, bell pepper, and carrot. Cook until vegetables are tender-crisp.

- Pour in soy sauce and hoisin sauce, tossing to coat.

- Serve over cooked brown rice.

Serving Methods:

1. Plate as a traditional stir-fry.

2. Wrap in lettuce leaves for a low-carb option.

Quinoa and Black Bean Stuffed Bell Peppers

Ingredients:

- 4 bell peppers, halved and seeds removed

- 1 cup cooked quinoa

- 1 can (15 oz) black beans, drained and rinsed

- 1 cup corn kernels

- 1/2 cup diced tomatoes

- 1 teaspoon cumin

- 1 teaspoon chili powder

- 1/4 cup shredded Monterey Jack cheese

Preparation Time: 20 minutes

Cooking Time: 25 minutes

Serving Time: 5 minutes

Nutritional Info: High in fiber, plant-based protein, and vitamins.

Instructions:

- Preheat the oven to 375°F (190°C).

- In a bowl, mix quinoa, black beans, corn, tomatoes, cumin, and chili powder.

- Stuff bell peppers with the quinoa mixture.

- Top with shredded Monterey Jack cheese and bake until peppers are tender.

Serving Methods:

1. Arrange as a colorful main course.

2. Slice into halves for a visually appealing side dish.

Chickpea and Spinach Curry

Ingredients:

- 1 can (15 oz.) chickpeas, drained and rinsed

- 2 cups fresh spinach leaves

- 1 onion, finely chopped

- 2 tomatoes, diced

- 2 cloves garlic, minced

- 1 tablespoon ginger, grated

- 1 tablespoon curry powder

- 1 can (13.5 oz.) coconut milk

Preparation Time: 15 minutes

Cooking Time: 20 minutes

Serving Time: 5 minutes

Nutritional Info: High in plant-based protein, iron, and vitamins.

Instructions:

- Sauté onions, garlic, and ginger until fragrant.

- Add chickpeas, tomatoes, and curry powder. Cook until tomatoes soften.

- Pour in coconut milk and simmer until flavors meld.

- Stir in fresh spinach until wilted.

Serving Methods:

1. Serve over basmati rice for a classic curry dish.

2. Spoon over roasted sweet potatoes for a twist.

Caprese Salad with Grilled Chicken

Ingredients:

- 200g chicken breast, grilled and sliced

- 2 cups cherry tomatoes, halved

- 1 cup fresh mozzarella balls

- 1 bunch fresh basil leaves

- 2 tablespoons balsamic glaze

- 2 tablespoons extra virgin olive oil

- Salt and pepper to taste

Preparation Time: 15 minutes

Cooking Time: 15 minutes

Serving Time: 5 minutes

Nutritional Info: High in protein, antioxidants, and healthy fats.

Instructions:

- Grill chicken until fully cooked. Slice into strips.

- In a bowl, combine cherry tomatoes, fresh mozzarella, and basil leaves.

- Drizzle with balsamic glaze and olive oil. Season with salt and pepper.

- Arrange grilled chicken on top.

Serving Methods:

1. Serve on a large platter for a shared lunch.

2. Assemble on skewers for a portable option.

Spinach and Mushroom Quiche

Ingredients:

- 1 ready-made whole-grain pie crust

- 2 cups fresh spinach, chopped

- 1 cup mushrooms, sliced

- 1 onion, diced

- 4 eggs

- 1 cup milk (dairy or plant-based)

- 1/2 cup shredded Swiss cheese

- Salt and pepper to taste

Preparation Time: 20 minutes

Cooking Time: 35 minutes

Serving Time: 5 minutes

Nutritional Info: High in vitamins, minerals, and protein.

Instructions:

- Preheat the oven to 375°F (190°C).

- Sauté mushrooms and onions until softened. Add spinach and cook until wilted.

- In a bowl, whisk eggs, milk, shredded Swiss cheese, salt, and pepper.

- Pour the egg mixture into the pie crust. Add the sautéed vegetables.

- Bake until the quiche is set and golden brown.

Serving Methods:

1. Serve slices on individual plates.

2. Cut into squares and serve as bite-sized portions.

Turkey and Quinoa Stuffed Zucchini Boats

Ingredients:

- 2 large zucchinis, halved lengthwise

- 200g lean ground turkey

- 1 cup cooked quinoa

- 1/2 cup diced tomatoes

- 1/4 cup black olives, sliced

- 1 teaspoon Italian seasoning

- 1/4 cup grated Parmesan cheese

Preparation Time: 20 minutes

Cooking Time: 25 minutes

Serving Time: 5 minutes

Nutritional Info: High in protein, fiber, and essential nutrients.

Instructions:

- Preheat the oven to 375°F (190°C).

- Scoop out the center of the zucchinis to create boats.

- Cook ground turkey until browned. Mix with quinoa, tomatoes, olives, and Italian seasoning.

- Stuff the zucchini boats with the turkey and quinoa mixture.

- Top with grated Parmesan cheese and bake until zucchini is tender.

Serving Methods:

1. Arrange zucchini boats on a plate.

2. Serve as a side dish for a larger meal.

Mango and Shrimp Salad

Ingredients:

- 200g shrimp, cooked and peeled

- 1 mango, diced

- 1 avocado, sliced

- 1 cup mixed greens (arugula, watercress)

- 2 tablespoons lime juice

- 1 tablespoon olive oil

- Salt and pepper to taste

Preparation Time: 15 minutes

Cooking Time: 5 minutes

Serving Time: 5 minutes

Nutritional Info: High in protein, vitamins, and healthy fats.

Instructions:

- In a bowl, combine shrimp, diced mango, avocado slices, and mixed greens.

- Drizzle with lime juice and olive oil. Season with salt and pepper.

- Toss gently to combine.

Serving Methods:

1. Serve in a large bowl for a refreshing salad.

2. Arrange on a flatbread for a tropical shrimp wrap.

Eggplant and Chickpea Buddha Bowl

Ingredients:

- 1 medium eggplant, diced

- 1 can (15 oz.) chickpeas, drained and rinsed

- 1 cup quinoa, cooked

- 1/2 cup cherry tomatoes, halved

- 1/4 cup tahini

- 2 tablespoons lemon juice

- 1 clove garlic, minced

- Fresh parsley for garnish

Preparation Time: 15 minutes

Cooking Time: 20 minutes

Serving Time: 5 minutes

Nutritional Info: High in fiber, plant-based protein, and antioxidants.

Instructions:

- Roast diced eggplant until golden brown. Sauté chickpeas until crisp.

- Assemble bowls with cooked quinoa, roasted eggplant, sautéed chickpeas, and cherry tomatoes.
- In a small bowl, mix tahini, lemon juice, and minced garlic. Drizzle over the bowls.
- Garnish with fresh parsley.

Serving Methods:

1. Serve in individual bowls.

2. Arrange ingredients on a platter for a communal Buddha bowl experience.

CHAPTER SEVEN

DINNER RECIPES

Grilled Lemon Herb Chicken

Ingredients:

- 4 boneless, skinless chicken breasts
- 2 tablespoons olive oil
- 1 lemon, juiced
- 2 cloves garlic, minced
- 1 teaspoon dried thyme
- 1 teaspoon dried rosemary
- Salt and pepper to taste

Preparation Time: 10 minutes

Cooking Time: 15 minutes

Serving Time: 5 minutes

Nutritional Info: High in protein, low in saturated fat.

Instructions:

- In a bowl, mix olive oil, lemon juice, garlic, thyme, rosemary, salt, and pepper.

- Marinate chicken breasts in the mixture for at least 30 minutes.

- Grill until fully cooked.

- Serve with a side of roasted vegetables or quinoa.

Serving Methods:

1. Slice chicken and serve on individual plates.

2. Shred chicken for tacos with whole-grain tortillas.

Baked Salmon with Dill Sauce

Ingredients:

- 4 salmon fillets

- 1 tablespoon olive oil

- 1 lemon, sliced

- 2 tablespoons fresh dill, chopped

- Salt and pepper to taste

Preparation Time: 10 minutes

Cooking Time: 20 minutes

Serving Time: 5 minutes

Nutritional Info: Rich in omega-3s, high-quality protein.

Instructions:

- Preheat the oven to 375°F (190°C).

- Place salmon fillets on a baking sheet.

- Drizzle with olive oil, sprinkle with chopped dill, and season with salt and pepper.

- Arrange lemon slices on top of each fillet.

- Bake until salmon is flaky.

- Serve with a side of steamed broccoli or a quinoa salad.

Serving Methods:

1. Serve whole fillets on plates.

2. Flake salmon and toss with pasta for a quick dinner.

Vegetable and Tofu Stir-Fry

Ingredients:

- 200g extra-firm tofu, cubed

- 2 cups broccoli florets

- 1 red bell pepper, sliced

- 1 carrot, julienned

- 2 tablespoons low-sodium soy sauce

- 1 tablespoon hoisin sauce

- 1 tablespoon sesame oil

- 1 cup brown rice, cooked

Preparation Time: 15 minutes

Cooking Time: 15 minutes

Serving Time: 5 minutes

Nutritional Info: High in plant-based protein, fiber.

Instructions:

- Press tofu to remove excess water, then cube.

- Sauté tofu in sesame oil until golden brown.

- Add broccoli, bell pepper, and carrot. Stir-fry until vegetables are tender-crisp.

- Pour in soy sauce and hoisin sauce. Toss to coat.

- Serve over cooked brown rice.

Serving Methods:

1. Plate as a traditional stir-fry.

2. Wrap in lettuce leaves for a low-carb option.

Mushroom and Spinach Stuffed Chicken Breast

Ingredients:

- 4 boneless, skinless chicken breasts

- 1 cup mushrooms, chopped

- 2 cups fresh spinach

- 1/2 cup feta cheese, crumbled

- 1 tablespoon olive oil

- Salt and pepper to taste

Preparation Time: 20 minutes

Cooking Time: 25 minutes

Serving Time: 5 minutes

Nutritional Info: High in protein, vitamins, and minerals.

Instructions:

- Preheat the oven to 375°F (190°C).

- Sauté mushrooms in olive oil until softened. Add spinach and cook until wilted.

- Slice a pocket into each chicken breast.

- Stuff each breast with the mushroom and spinach mixture and crumbled feta.

- Season with salt and pepper.

- Bake until chicken is cooked through.

- Serve with a side of roasted sweet potatoes or quinoa.

Serving Methods:

1. Serve whole stuffed breasts on plates.

2. Slice and arrange on a platter for sharing.

Vegetarian Chili with Quinoa

Ingredients:

- 1 cup quinoa, cooked

- 1 can (15 oz.) black beans, drained and rinsed

- 1 can (15 oz.) kidney beans, drained and rinsed

- 1 can (15 oz.) diced tomatoes

- 1 cup corn kernels

- 1 onion, diced

- 2 cloves garlic, minced

- 1 tablespoon chili powder

- 1 teaspoon cumin

- Salt and pepper to taste

Preparation Time: 15 minutes

Cooking Time: 30 minutes

Serving Time: 5 minutes

Nutritional Info: High in protein, fiber, and essential nutrients.

Instructions:

- Sauté onions and garlic until softened.

- Add diced tomatoes, black beans, kidney beans, corn, chili powder, and cumin.

- Simmer until flavors meld.

- Serve over cooked quinoa.

- Garnish with cilantro and a dollop of Greek yogurt.

Serving Methods:

1. Ladle into bowls for a cozy dinner.

2. Spoon over baked sweet potatoes for a twist.

Lemon Garlic Shrimp Pasta

Ingredients:

- 200g shrimp, peeled and deveined

- 8 oz. whole-grain spaghetti

- 2 tablespoons olive oil

- 3 cloves garlic, minced

- 1 lemon, zested and juiced

- 1/4 cup fresh parsley, chopped

- Salt and pepper to taste

- Grated Parmesan cheese for topping

Preparation Time: 15 minutes

Cooking Time: 15 minutes

Serving Time: 5 minutes

Nutritional Info: High in protein, whole grains, and healthy fats.

Instructions:

- Cook pasta according to package instructions.

- Sauté shrimp in olive oil with minced garlic until pink.

- Toss cooked pasta with shrimp, lemon zest, lemon juice, and chopped parsley.

- Season with salt and pepper.

- Top with grated Parmesan cheese.

Serving Methods:

1. Plate individual servings.

2. Serve in a large bowl for a family-style dinner.

Quinoa and Vegetable Stuffed Bell Peppers

Ingredients:

- 4 bell peppers, halved and seeds removed
- 1 cup cooked quinoa
- 1 cup black beans, drained and rinsed
- 1 cup corn kernels
- 1/2 cup diced tomatoes
- 1/2 cup shredded cheddar cheese
- 1 teaspoon cumin
- 1 teaspoon chili powder
- Fresh cilantro for garnish

Preparation Time: 20 minutes

Cooking Time: 25 minutes

Serving Time: 5 minutes

Nutritional Info: High in fiber, plant-based protein, and vitamins.

Instructions:

- Preheat the oven to 375°F (190°C).

- In a bowl, mix quinoa, black beans, corn, tomatoes, shredded cheddar, cumin, and chili powder.

- Stuff bell peppers with the quinoa mixture.

- Bake until peppers are tender.

- Garnish with fresh cilantro.

Serving Methods:

1. Arrange as a colorful main course.

2. Slice into halves for a visually appealing side dish.

Teriyaki Tofu and Broccoli Stir-Fry

Ingredients:

- 200g firm tofu, cubed

- 2 cups broccoli florets

- 1 bell pepper, sliced

- 1/4 cup low-sodium teriyaki sauce

- 1 tablespoon sesame oil

- 2 tablespoons green onions, chopped

- Sesame seeds for garnish

- Brown rice for serving

Preparation Time: 15 minutes

Cooking Time: 15 minutes

Serving Time: 5 minutes

Nutritional Info: High in plant-based protein, fiber, and essential nutrients

Instructions:

- Sauté tofu in sesame oil until golden brown.

- Add broccoli and bell pepper. Stir-fry until vegetables are tender-crisp.

- Pour in teriyaki sauce, tossing to coat.

- Serve over cooked brown rice.

- Garnish with chopped green onions and sesame seeds.

Serving Methods:

1. Plate as a traditional stir-fry.

2. Roll the stir-fry in lettuce leaves for a low-carb option.

Mediterranean Chickpea and Spinach Stew

Ingredients:

- 1 can (15 oz.) chickpeas, drained and rinsed

- 4 cups fresh spinach

- 1 onion, diced

- 2 tomatoes, diced

- 3 cloves garlic, minced

- 1 teaspoon cumin

- 1 teaspoon smoked paprika

- 1/4 cup fresh parsley, chopped

Preparation Time: 15 minutes

Cooking Time: 20 minutes

Serving Time: 5 minutes

Nutritional Info: High in fiber, plant-based protein, and antioxidants.

Instructions:

- Sauté onions and garlic until softened.

- Add chickpeas, tomatoes, cumin, and smoked paprika. Cook until tomatoes soften.

- Stir in fresh spinach until wilted.

- Garnish with fresh parsley before serving.

- Serve with a side of whole-grain bread or couscous.

Serving Methods:

1. Ladle into bowls for a comforting stew.

2. Spoon over quinoa for a protein-packed dinner.

Baked Eggplant Parmesan

Ingredients:

- 1 large eggplant, sliced

- 1 cup whole wheat breadcrumbs

- 2 eggs, beaten

- 2 cups marinara sauce

- 1 cup mozzarella cheese, shredded

- 1/4 cup Parmesan cheese, grated

- Fresh basil for garnish

Preparation Time: 20 minutes

Cooking Time: 25 minutes

Serving Time: 5 minutes

Nutritional Info: High in fiber, vitamins, and minerals.

Instructions:

- Preheat the oven to 375°F (190°C).

- Dip eggplant slices in beaten eggs, then coat with breadcrumbs.

- Arrange on a baking sheet and bake until golden brown.

- In a baking dish, layer marinara sauce, baked eggplant, and cheeses.

- Bake until cheese is melted and bubbly.

- Garnish with fresh basil before serving.

Serving Methods:

1. Serve individual portions on plates.

2. Layer between whole-grain bread for an eggplant Parmesan sandwich.

Lemon Garlic Herb Baked Cod

Ingredients:

- 4 cod fillets

- 2 tablespoons olive oil

- 2 cloves garlic, minced

- 1 lemon, juiced and zested

*   1 teaspoon dried thyme

*   Salt and pepper to taste

Preparation Time: 10 minutes

Cooking Time: 15 minutes

Serving Time: 5 minutes

Nutritional Info: High in lean protein, omega-3s, and vitamin C.

Instructions:

*   Preheat the oven to 400°F (200°C).

*   Place cod fillets on a baking sheet.

*   Mix olive oil, minced garlic, lemon juice, lemon zest, thyme, salt, and pepper.

*   Brush the mixture over the cod fillets.

*   Bake until the fish is flaky.

*   Serve with roasted vegetables or a side salad.

Serving Methods:

1. Plate individual fillets.

2. Serve over quinoa for a heartier meal.

Chicken and Vegetable Skewers with Peanut Sauce

Ingredients:

- 2 boneless, skinless chicken breasts, cubed

- 1 zucchini, sliced

- 1 bell pepper, cut into chunks

- 1/4 cup low-sodium soy sauce

- 2 tablespoons peanut butter

- 1 tablespoon honey

- 1 teaspoon ginger, grated

- Wooden skewers, soaked in water

Preparation Time: 20 minutes

Cooking Time: 15 minutes

Serving Time: 5 minutes

Nutritional Info: Balanced protein, vegetables, and healthy fats.

Instructions:

- Preheat the grill or grill pan.

- Thread chicken, zucchini, and bell pepper onto skewers.

- In a bowl, whisk soy sauce, peanut butter, honey, and ginger for the sauce.

- Grill skewers until chicken is cooked.

- Serve with brown rice or quinoa.

- Drizzle peanut sauce over the skewers.

Serving Methods:

1. Arrange skewers on a plate.

2. Serve over a bed of mixed greens for a salad.

Turmeric and Coconut Curry with Shrimp

Ingredients:

- 200g shrimp, peeled and deveined

- 1 onion, diced

- 2 cloves garlic, minced

- 1 tablespoon ginger, grated

- 1 can (13.5 oz) coconut milk

- 1 tablespoon curry powder

- 1 teaspoon turmeric

- 1 cup broccoli florets

- Fresh cilantro for garnish

- Brown rice for serving

Preparation Time: 15 minutes

Cooking Time: 20 minutes

Serving Time: 5 minutes

Nutritional Info: Rich in omega-3s, anti-inflammatory.

Instructions:

- Sauté onions, garlic, and ginger until fragrant.

- Add shrimp and cook until pink.

- Stir in curry powder and turmeric.

- Pour in coconut milk and simmer.

- Add broccoli and cook until tender.

- Serve over brown rice.

- Garnish with fresh cilantro.

Serving Methods:

1. Plate curry over rice.

2. Spoon into lettuce leaves for a carb-free option.

Quinoa and Black Bean Stuffed Acorn Squash

Ingredients:

- 2 acorn squash, halved and seeds removed

- 1 cup cooked quinoa

- 1 can (15 oz.) black beans, drained and rinsed

- 1 cup cherry tomatoes, halved

- 1/2 cup red onion, finely chopped

- 1 teaspoon cumin

- 1 teaspoon chili powder

- 1/4 cup feta cheese, crumbled

Preparation Time: 20 minutes

Cooking Time: 30 minutes

Serving Time: 5 minutes

Nutritional Info: High in fiber, plant-based protein, and vitamins.

Instructions:

- Preheat the oven to 375°F (190°C).

- Place acorn squash halves on a baking sheet.

- In a bowl, mix quinoa, black beans, cherry tomatoes, red onion, cumin, and chili powder.

- Stuff acorn squash with the quinoa mixture.

- Top with crumbled feta cheese.

- Bake until squash is tender.

- Serve with a side of mixed greens.

Serving Methods:

1. Plate stuffed squash halves.

2. Cut into quarters for a visually appealing side dish.

Salmon and Asparagus Foil Packets

Ingredients:

- 4 salmon fillets

- 1 bunch asparagus, trimmed

- 2 tablespoons olive oil

- 1 lemon, sliced

- 2 cloves garlic, minced

- Salt and pepper to taste

Preparation Time: 15 minutes

Cooking Time: 20 minutes

Serving Time: 5 minutes

Nutritional Info: Omega-3s, antioxidants, and vitamin C.

Instructions:

- Preheat the oven to 400°F (200°C).

- Place each salmon fillet on a piece of foil.

- Arrange asparagus around the salmon.

- Drizzle with olive oil, sprinkle minced garlic, and season with salt and pepper.

- Place lemon slices on top.

- Seal the foil packets and bake until salmon is cooked.

- Serve with a side of quinoa or wild rice.

Serving Methods:

1. Serve in the foil for easy cleanup.

2. Plate individually with a lemon wedge.

Vegetarian Lentil and Vegetable Stew

Ingredients:

- 1 cup dried green lentils

- 1 onion, diced

- 2 carrots, chopped

- 2 celery stalks, sliced

- 1 cup butternut squash, diced

- 1 can (15 oz.) diced tomatoes

- 4 cups vegetable broth

- 1 teaspoon cumin

- 1 teaspoon smoked paprika

- Salt and pepper to taste

Preparation Time: 15 minutes

Cooking Time: 30 minutes

Serving Time: 5 minutes

Nutritional Info: High in protein, fiber, and antioxidants.

Instructions:

- Rinse lentils and cook in vegetable broth until tender.

- Sauté onions, carrots, and celery until softened.

- Add butternut squash, diced tomatoes, cumin, smoked paprika, salt, and pepper.

- Combine sautéed vegetables with cooked lentils.

- Simmer until flavors meld.

- Serve with a slice of whole-grain bread.

Serving Methods:

1. Ladle into bowls for a comforting stew.

2. Spoon over brown rice for a heartier meal.

Mushroom and Spinach Brown Rice Risotto

Ingredients:

- 1 cup brown rice, cooked

- 1 cup mushrooms, sliced

- 2 cups fresh spinach

- 1 onion, diced

- 2 cloves garlic, minced

- 1/2 cup Parmesan cheese, grated

- 2 tablespoons olive oil

- Salt and pepper to taste

Preparation Time: 20 minutes

Cooking Time: 25 minutes

Serving Time: 5 minutes

Nutritional Info: High in fiber, vitamins, and minerals.

Instructions:

- Sauté onions and garlic in olive oil until softened.

- Add mushrooms and cook until browned.

- Stir in fresh spinach until wilted.

- Mix in cooked brown rice and Parmesan cheese.

- Season with salt and pepper.

- Serve with a side of steamed broccoli or a green salad.

Serving Methods:

1. Plate as a side dish.

2. Serve as a main course with a protein source.

Sweet Potato and Turkey Skillet

Ingredients:

- 1 lb. ground turkey

- 2 sweet potatoes, peeled and diced

- 1 bell pepper, diced

- 1 onion, chopped

- 2 tablespoons olive oil

- 1 teaspoon ground cumin

- 1 teaspoon smoked paprika

- Salt and pepper to taste

Preparation Time: 15 minutes

Cooking Time: 20 minutes

Serving Time: 5 minutes

Nutritional Info: Lean protein, beta-carotene, and fiber.

Instructions:

- In a skillet, heat olive oil and sauté onions until translucent.

- Add ground turkey and cook until browned.

- Stir in sweet potatoes, bell pepper, cumin, smoked paprika, salt, and pepper.

- Cook until sweet potatoes are tender.

- Serve with a side of quinoa or whole-grain couscous.

Serving Methods:

1. Serve in the skillet for a rustic presentation.

2. Plate over a bed of greens for a lighter option.

Chickpea and Vegetable Coconut Curry

Ingredients:

- 1 can (15 oz.) chickpeas, drained and rinsed

- 1 cup broccoli florets

- 1 bell pepper, sliced

- 1 carrot, julienned

- 1 can (13.5 oz) coconut milk

- 2 tablespoons red curry paste

- 1 tablespoon soy sauce

- Fresh cilantro for garnish

- Basmati rice for serving

Preparation Time: 15 minutes

Cooking Time: 20 minutes

Serving Time: 5 minutes

Nutritional Info: Plant-based protein, vitamins, and healthy fats.

Instructions:

- Sauté broccoli, bell pepper, and carrot until slightly tender.

- Stir in chickpeas, red curry paste, and soy sauce.

- Pour in coconut milk and simmer until vegetables are cooked.

- Serve over basmati rice.

- Garnish with fresh cilantro.

Serving Methods:

1. Ladle into bowls for a comforting curry.

2. Spoon over quinoa for a protein boost.

Spinach and Feta Stuffed Chicken Thighs

Ingredients:

- 4 bone-in, skin-on chicken thighs

- 2 cups fresh spinach

- 1/2 cup feta cheese, crumbled

- 1 lemon, zested and juiced

- 2 cloves garlic, minced

- 1 tablespoon olive oil

- Salt and pepper to taste

Preparation Time: 15 minutes

Cooking Time: 20 minutes

Serving Time: 5 minutes

Nutritional Info: Plant-based protein, vitamins, and healthy fats

Instructions:

- Preheat the oven to 375°F (190°C).

- Create a pocket in each chicken thigh by gently lifting the skin.

- In a bowl, mix fresh spinach, feta cheese, lemon zest, lemon juice, minced garlic, salt, and pepper.

- Stuff each thigh with the spinach and feta mixture.

- Drizzle olive oil over the chicken.

- Bake until chicken is cooked through and skin is crispy.

- Serve with a side of roasted vegetables or a green salad.

Serving Methods:

1. Place stuffed thighs on individual plates.

2. Arrange on a platter for a family-style presentation.

CHAPTER EIGHT

SNACKS RECIPES

Lemon Herb Grilled Salmon

Ingredients:

- 4 salmon fillets

- 2 tablespoons olive oil

- 1 lemon, juiced and zested

- 2 cloves garlic, minced

- 1 teaspoon dried thyme

- Salt and pepper to taste

Preparation Time: 15 minutes

Grilling Time: 10 minutes

Serving Time: 5 minutes

Nutritional Info: Omega-3s, lean protein, and vitamin C.

Instructions:

- In a bowl, mix olive oil, lemon juice, lemon zest, minced garlic, dried thyme, salt, and pepper.

- Marinate salmon fillets in the mixture for at least 10 minutes.

- Grill salmon until it flakes easily.

- Serve with a side of quinoa or roasted vegetables.

Serving Methods:

1. Plate individual fillets.

2. Serve over a bed of steamed spinach for a vibrant dish.

Vegetarian Stuffed Bell Peppers

Ingredients:

- 4 bell peppers, halved and seeds removed

- 1 cup cooked quinoa

- 1 can (15 oz.) black beans, drained and rinsed

- 1 cup corn kernels

- 1 cup diced tomatoes

- 1 teaspoon cumin

- 1 teaspoon chili powder

- Shredded cheddar cheese for topping

Preparation Time: 20 minutes

Baking Time: 25 minutes

Serving Time: 5 minutes

Nutritional Info: Fiber, plant-based protein, and antioxidants.

Instructions:

- Preheat the oven to 375°F (190°C).

- In a bowl, mix quinoa, black beans, corn, tomatoes, cumin, and chili powder.

- Stuff bell peppers with the quinoa mixture.

- Bake until peppers are tender.

- Top with shredded cheddar cheese.

- Garnish with fresh cilantro.

Serving Methods:

1. Arrange as a colorful main course.

2. Slice into halves for a visually appealing side dish.

Teriyaki Tofu and Broccoli Stir-Fry

Ingredients:

- 200g firm tofu, cubed

- 2 cups broccoli florets

- 1 bell pepper, sliced

- 1/4 cup low-sodium teriyaki sauce

- 1 tablespoon sesame oil

- 2 tablespoons green onions, chopped

- Sesame seeds for garnish

- Brown rice for serving

Preparation Time: 15 minutes

Cooking Time: 15 minutes

Serving Time: 5 minutes

Nutritional Info: Plant-based protein, fiber, and essential nutrients.

Instructions:

- Sauté tofu in sesame oil until golden brown.

- Add broccoli and bell pepper. Stir-fry until vegetables are tender-crisp.

- Pour in teriyaki sauce, tossing to coat.

- Serve over cooked brown rice.

- Garnish with chopped green onions and sesame seeds.

Serving Methods:

1. Plate as a traditional stir-fry.

2. Roll the stir-fry in lettuce leaves for a low-carb option.

Mediterranean Chickpea and Spinach Stew

Ingredients:

- 1 can (15 oz.) chickpeas, drained and rinsed
- 4 cups fresh spinach
- 1 onion, diced
- 2 tomatoes, diced
- 3 cloves garlic, minced
- 1 teaspoon cumin
- 1 teaspoon smoked paprika
- 1/4 cup fresh parsley, chopped

Preparation Time: 15 minutes

Cooking Time: 20 minutes

Serving Time: 5 minutes

Nutritional Info: Fiber, plant-based protein, and antioxidants.

Instructions:

- Sauté onions and garlic until softened.

- Add chickpeas, tomatoes, cumin, and smoked paprika. Cook until tomatoes soften.

- Stir in fresh spinach until wilted.

- Garnish with fresh parsley before serving.

- Serve with a side of whole-grain bread or couscous.

Serving Methods:

1. Ladle into bowls for a comforting stew.

2. Spoon over quinoa for a protein-packed dinner.

Baked Eggplant Parmesan

Ingredients:

- 1 large eggplant, sliced

- 1 cup whole wheat breadcrumbs

- 2 eggs, beaten

- 2 cups marinara sauce

- 1 cup mozzarella cheese, shredded

- 1/4 cup Parmesan cheese, grated

- Fresh basil for garnish

Preparation Time: 20 minutes

Baking Time: 25 minutes

Serving Time: 5 minutes

Nutritional Info: Fiber, vitamins, and minerals.

Instructions:

- Preheat the oven to 375°F (190°C).

- Dip eggplant slices in beaten eggs, then coat with breadcrumbs.

- Arrange on a baking sheet and bake until golden brown.

- In a baking dish, layer marinara sauce, baked eggplant, and cheeses.

- Bake until cheese is melted and bubbly.

- Garnish with fresh basil before serving.

Serving Methods:

1. Serve individual portions on plates.

2. Layer between whole-grain bread for an eggplant Parmesan sandwich.

Lemon Garlic Herb Grilled Chicken

Ingredients:

- 4 boneless, skinless chicken breasts

- 2 tablespoons olive oil

- 3 cloves garlic, minced

- 1 lemon, juiced and zested

- 1 teaspoon dried oregano

- Salt and pepper to taste

Preparation Time: 15 minutes

Grilling Time: 15 minutes

Serving Time: 5 minutes

Nutritional Info: Lean protein, vitamin C, and antioxidants.

Instructions:

- In a bowl, mix olive oil, minced garlic, lemon juice, lemon zest, dried oregano, salt, and pepper.

- Marinate chicken breasts in the mixture for at least 30 minutes.

- Grill chicken until fully cooked.

- Serve with a side of quinoa or roasted sweet potatoes.

Serving Methods:

- Plate individual chicken breasts.

- Slice and arrange on a platter for a family-style presentation.

Chickpea and Vegetable Coconut Curry

Ingredients:

- 1 can (15 oz.) chickpeas, drained and rinsed

- 1 cup broccoli florets

- 1 bell pepper, sliced

- 1 carrot, julienned

- 1 can (13.5 oz.) coconut milk

- 2 tablespoons red curry paste

- 1 tablespoon soy sauce

- Fresh cilantro for garnish

- Basmati rice for serving

Preparation Time: 15 minutes

Cooking Time: 20 minutes

Serving Time: 5 minutes

Nutritional Info: Plant-based protein, vitamins, and healthy fats.

Instructions:

- Sauté broccoli, bell pepper, and carrot until slightly tender.

- Stir in chickpeas, red curry paste, and soy sauce.

- Pour in coconut milk and simmer until vegetables are cooked.

- Serve over basmati rice.

- Garnish with fresh cilantro.

Serving Methods:

1. Ladle into bowls for a comforting curry.

2. Spoon over quinoa for a protein boost.

Turkey and Vegetable Skillet with Quinoa

Ingredients:

- 1 lb. ground turkey

- 1 zucchini, diced

- 1 bell pepper, diced

- 1 cup cherry tomatoes, halved

- 1 cup cooked quinoa

- 2 tablespoons olive oil

- 1 teaspoon Italian seasoning

- Salt and pepper to taste

Preparation Time: 15 minutes

Cooking Time: 20 minutes

Serving Time: 5 minutes

Nutritional Info: Lean protein, fiber, and essential nutrients.

Instructions:

- In a skillet, heat olive oil and brown ground turkey.

- Add diced zucchini, bell pepper, and cherry tomatoes. Sauté until vegetables are tender.

- Stir in cooked quinoa and Italian seasoning.

- Season with salt and pepper.

- Serve with a sprinkle of fresh parsley.

Serving Methods:

1. Serve in the skillet for a rustic presentation.

2. Plate over a bed of mixed greens for a lighter option.

Miso-Glazed Cod with Stir-Fried Vegetables

Ingredients:

- 4 cod fillets

- 2 tablespoons white miso paste

- 1 tablespoon soy sauce

- 1 tablespoon mirin

- 1 tablespoon sesame oil

- 1 cup snap peas

- 1 cup bok choy, chopped

- 1 carrot, julienned

- Brown rice for serving

Preparation Time: 20 minutes

Cooking Time: 15 minutes

Serving Time: 5 minutes

Nutritional Info: Omega-3s, protein, and antioxidants.

Instructions:

- Preheat the oven to 400°F (200°C).

- Mix miso paste, soy sauce, mirin, and sesame oil to create the glaze.

- Brush cod fillets with the miso glaze and bake until cooked through.

- Stir-fry snap peas, bok choy, and julienned carrot in a hot pan.

- Serve cod over brown rice with the stir-fried vegetables.

Serving Methods:

1. Plate individual portions.

2. Arrange on a platter for a family-style dinner.

Quinoa and Lentil Stuffed Acorn Squash

Ingredients:

- 2 acorn squash, halved and seeds removed

- 1 cup cooked quinoa

- 1 cup cooked lentils

- 1/2 cup cranberries, dried

- 1/4 cup pecans, chopped

- 1 tablespoon maple syrup

- 1 teaspoon cinnamon

Preparation Time: 20 minutes

Baking Time: 30 minutes

Serving Time: 5 minutes

Nutritional Info: Fiber, plant-based protein, and antioxidants.

Instructions:

- Preheat the oven to 375°F (190°C).

- Place acorn squash halves on a baking sheet.

- In a bowl, mix cooked quinoa, cooked lentils, dried cranberries, chopped pecans, maple syrup, and cinnamon.

- Stuff acorn squash with the quinoa and lentil mixture.

- Bake until squash is tender.

- Serve with a drizzle of additional maple syrup.

Serving Methods:

1. Plate stuffed squash halves.

2. Cut into quarters for a visually appealing side dish.

Salmon and Asparagus Foil Packets

Ingredients:

- 4 salmon fillets

- 1 bunch asparagus, trimmed

- 2 tablespoons olive oil

- 1 lemon, sliced

- 2 cloves garlic, minced

- Fresh dill for garnish

- Salt and pepper to taste

Preparation Time: 15 minutes

Baking Time: 20 minutes

Serving Time: 5 minutes

Nutritional Info: Omega-3s, vitamins, and antioxidants.

Instructions:

- Preheat the oven to 400°F (200°C).

- Place each salmon fillet on a piece of foil.

- Arrange asparagus around the salmon.

- Drizzle with olive oil, sprinkle minced garlic, and season with salt and pepper.

- Top with lemon slices and seal the foil packets.

- Bake until salmon is cooked through.

- Garnish with fresh dill before serving.

Serving Methods:

1. Serve individual foil packets.

2. Plate over a bed of quinoa for a complete meal.

Shrimp and Vegetable Stir-Fry

Ingredients:

- 1 lb. shrimp, peeled and deveined

- 2 cups broccoli florets

- 1 bell pepper, sliced

- 1 cup snow peas

- 2 tablespoons soy sauce

- 1 tablespoon sesame oil

- 1 teaspoon ginger, minced

- Brown rice for serving

Preparation Time: 15 minutes

Cooking Time: 10 minutes

Serving Time: 5 minutes

Nutritional Info: Lean protein, fiber, and essential nutrients.

Instructions:

- In a wok or skillet, heat sesame oil and sauté shrimp until pink.

- Add broccoli, bell pepper, and snow peas. Stir-fry until vegetables are tender-crisp.

- Stir in soy sauce and minced ginger.

- Serve over cooked brown rice.

Serving Methods:

1. Plate individual servings.

2. Serve family-style in the wok for sharing.

Quinoa and Black Bean Stuffed Peppers

Ingredients:

- 4 bell peppers, halved and seeds removed

- 1 cup cooked quinoa

- 1 can (15 oz.) black beans, drained and rinsed

- 1 cup corn kernels

- 1 cup diced tomatoes

- 1 teaspoon cumin

- 1 teaspoon chili powder

- Guacamole for topping

Preparation Time: 20 minutes

Baking Time: 25 minutes

Serving Time: 5 minutes

Nutritional Info: Fiber, plant-based protein, and antioxidants.

Instructions:

- Preheat the oven to 375°F (190°C).

- In a bowl, mix quinoa, black beans, corn, tomatoes, cumin, and chili powder.

- Stuff bell peppers with the quinoa mixture.

- Bake until peppers are tender.

- Top with guacamole before serving.

Serving Methods:

1. Arrange as a colorful main course.

2. Slice into halves for a visually appealing side dish.

Chicken and Vegetable Skewers with Tzatziki Sauce

Ingredients:

- 1 lb. chicken breast, cut into cubes

- 1 zucchini, sliced

- 1 bell pepper, cut into chunks

- 1 red onion, cut into wedges

- 1/4 cup olive oil

- 1 teaspoon oregano

- Salt and pepper to taste

- Tzatziki sauce for dipping

Preparation Time: 20 minutes

Grilling Time: 15 minutes

Serving Time: 5 minutes

Nutritional Info: Lean protein, vitamins, and healthy fats.

Instructions:

- Preheat the grill to medium-high heat.

- Thread chicken and vegetables onto skewers.

- In a bowl, mix olive oil, oregano, salt, and pepper.

- Brush skewers with the olive oil mixture.

- Grill until chicken is cooked through.

- Serve with tzatziki sauce for dipping.

Serving Methods:

1. Serve on individual plates.

2. Arrange on a platter for a shared appetizer.

Vegetarian Lentil and Sweet Potato Curry

Ingredients:

- 1 cup dry green lentils, rinsed

- 2 sweet potatoes, peeled and diced

- 1 can (14 oz.) diced tomatoes

- 1 can (13.5 oz.) coconut milk

- 1 onion, diced

- 2 cloves garlic, minced

- 1 tablespoon curry powder

- Fresh cilantro for garnish

- Basmati rice for serving

Preparation Time: 20 minutes

Cooking Time: 25 minutes

Serving Time: 5 minutes

Nutritional Info: Plant-based protein, fiber, and vitamins.

Instructions:

- In a pot, sauté onions and garlic until softened.

- Add lentils, sweet potatoes, diced tomatoes, coconut milk, and curry powder.

- Simmer until lentils and sweet potatoes are tender.

- Garnish with fresh cilantro.

- Serve over basmati rice.

Serving Methods:

1. Ladle into bowls for a comforting curry.

2. Spoon over quinoa for a protein boost.

Mushroom and Spinach Stuffed Chicken Breast

Ingredients:

- 4 boneless, skinless chicken breasts

- 2 cups mushrooms, chopped

- 2 cups fresh spinach

- 1/2 cup feta cheese, crumbled

- 2 tablespoons olive oil

- 2 cloves garlic, minced

- Salt and pepper to taste

Preparation Time: 20 minutes

Baking Time: 25 minutes

Serving Time: 5 minutes

Nutritional Info: Protein, iron, and vitamins.

Instructions:

- Preheat the oven to 375°F (190°C).

- In a skillet, sauté mushrooms and garlic in olive oil until softened.

- Add fresh spinach and cook until wilted.

- Remove from heat and stir in crumbled feta.

- Create a pocket in each chicken breast and stuff with the mushroom and spinach mixture.

- Bake until chicken is cooked through.

- Serve with a side of roasted vegetables.

Serving Methods:

1. Place stuffed chicken breasts on individual plates.

2. Arrange on a platter for a family-style presentation.

Cauliflower and Chickpea Buddha Bowl

Ingredients:

- 1 head cauliflower, cut into florets

- 1 can (15 oz.) chickpeas, drained and rinsed

- 2 tablespoons olive oil

- 1 teaspoon cumin

- 1 teaspoon smoked paprika

- Quinoa for serving

- Avocado slices for topping

- Tahini dressing

Preparation Time: 20 minutes

Roasting Time: 25 minutes

Serving Time: 5 minutes

Nutritional Info: Fiber, plant-based protein, and healthy fats.

Instructions:

- Preheat the oven to 400°F (200°C).

- Toss cauliflower florets and chickpeas with olive oil, cumin, and smoked paprika.

- Roast until cauliflower is golden brown.

- Serve over quinoa.

- Top with avocado slices.

- Drizzle with tahini dressing before serving.

Serving Methods:

1. Plate individual bowls.

2. Arrange components separately for a customizable bowl.

Turkey and Vegetable Chili

Ingredients:

- 1 lb. ground turkey

- 1 onion, diced

- 2 bell peppers, diced

- 2 cans (15 oz. each) kidney beans, drained and rinsed

- 1 can (28 oz.) crushed tomatoes

- 2 tablespoons chili powder

- 1 teaspoon cumin

- Sour cream and chopped green onions for topping

Preparation Time: 20 minutes

Cooking Time: 30 minutes

Serving Time: 5 minutes

Nutritional Info: Lean protein, fiber, and antioxidants.

Instructions:

- In a pot, brown ground turkey and onions.

- Add diced bell peppers, kidney beans, crushed tomatoes, chili powder, and cumin.

- Simmer until flavors meld.

- Serve with a dollop of sour cream and a sprinkle of chopped green onions.

Serving Methods:

1. Ladle into bowls for a comforting chili.

2. Spoon over baked sweet potatoes for a unique twist.

Pesto Zoodles with Grilled Chicken

Ingredients:

- 4 zucchinis, spiralized

- 1 lb. chicken breasts

- 1/2 cup cherry tomatoes, halved

- 1/4 cup pine nuts, toasted

- 1/2 cup basil pesto

- Parmesan cheese for topping

Preparation Time: 15 minutes

Grilling Time: 15 minutes

Serving Time: 5 minutes

Nutritional Info: Lean protein, vitamins, and healthy fats.

Instructions:

- Grill chicken breasts until fully cooked.

- Spiralize zucchinis to create zoodles.

- Toss zoodles with cherry tomatoes and toasted pine nuts.

- Slice grilled chicken and arrange over zoodles.

- Drizzle with basil pesto.

- Top with Parmesan cheese before serving.

Serving Methods:

1. Serve on individual plates.

2. Mix all components in a large bowl for a shared dish.

Spaghetti Squash with Turkey Bolognese

Ingredients:

- 1 large spaghetti squash, halved and seeds removed

- 1 lb. ground turkey

- 1 onion, diced

- 2 cloves garlic, minced

- 1 can (28 oz.) crushed tomatoes

- 1 teaspoon dried oregano

- 1 teaspoon dried basil

- Fresh parsley for garnish

Preparation Time: 20 minutes

Baking Time: 40 minutes

Serving Time: 5 minutes

Nutritional Info: Lean protein, vitamins, and fiber.

Instructions:

- Preheat the oven to 375°F (190°C).

- Place spaghetti squash halves on a baking sheet.

- In a skillet, brown ground turkey with diced onion and minced garlic.

- Add crushed tomatoes, oregano, and basil. Simmer until flavors meld.

- Use a fork to shred the cooked spaghetti squash into strands.

- Top with turkey Bolognese sauce.

- Garnish with fresh parsley before serving.

Serving Methods:

1. Plate individual portions.

2. Serve in the spaghetti squash shells for a creative presentation.

CHAPTER NINE

SNACKS RECIPES

Almond and Date Energy Bites

Ingredients:

- 1 cup almonds, toasted

- 1 cup pitted dates

- 1 tablespoon chia seeds

- 1 teaspoon vanilla extract

- Pinch of salt

- Shredded coconut for rolling

Preparation Time: 15 minutes

Serving Time: 5 minutes

Nutritional Info: Protein, fiber, and natural sugars.

Instructions:

- In a food processor, blend almonds, dates, chia seeds, vanilla extract, and salt until a sticky dough forms.

- Roll the mixture into bite-sized balls.

- Roll each ball in shredded coconut.

- Refrigerate for at least 30 minutes before serving.

Serving Methods:

1. Arrange on a plate for individual servings.

2. Pack in small containers for on-the-go snacking.

Greek Yogurt and Berry Parfait

Ingredients:

- 1 cup Greek yogurt

- 1/2 cup mixed berries (strawberries, blueberries, raspberries)

- 2 tablespoons honey

- Granola for topping

Preparation Time: 5 minutes

Serving Time: 5 minutes

Nutritional Info: Protein, probiotics, and antioxidants.

Instructions:

- In a glass or bowl, layer Greek yogurt and mixed berries.

- Drizzle honey over the layers.

- Top with granola for added crunch.

- Repeat the layers.

- Serve immediately.

Serving Methods:

1. Use clear glasses for an aesthetically pleasing presentation.

2. Mix all ingredients in a portable container for a snack on the move.

Cucumber and Hummus Bites

Ingredients:

- 1 cucumber, sliced

- 1/2 cup hummus

- Cherry tomatoes for topping

- Fresh parsley for garnish

Preparation Time: 10 minutes

Serving Time: 5 minutes

Nutritional Info: Fiber, healthy fats, and vitamins.

Instructions:

- Spread a small amount of hummus on each cucumber slice.

- Top with a halved cherry tomato.

- Garnish with fresh parsley.

- Arrange on a serving platter.

Serving Methods:

- Serve on a decorative platter for a party.

- Arrange on a plate for an individual snack.

Trail Mix with Dried Fruits and Nuts

Ingredients:

- 1 cup mixed nuts (almonds, walnuts, cashews)

- 1/2 cup dried apricots, chopped

- 1/2 cup dried cranberries

- 1/4 cup dark chocolate chips

- 1/4 teaspoon sea salt

Preparation Time: 5 minutes

Serving Time: 5 minutes

Nutritional Info: Protein, healthy fats, and antioxidants.

Instructions:

- In a bowl, mix together nuts, dried apricots, dried cranberries, dark chocolate chips, and sea salt.

- Toss until well combined.

- Portion into small snack-sized bags.

- Serve as needed.

Serving Methods:

1. Hand out individual bags for a quick grab-and-go snack.

2. Display on a serving tray for a shared snacking experience.

Apple Slices with Almond Butter

Ingredients:

- 2 apples, sliced

- 1/4 cup almond butter

- Cinnamon for sprinkling

Preparation Time: 5 minutes

Serving Time: 5 minutes

Nutritional Info: Fiber, protein, and natural sugars.

Instructions:

- Spread almond butter on apple slices.

- Sprinkle with cinnamon.

- Arrange on a plate for serving.

Serving Methods:

1. Arrange slices on a plate for an individual snack.

2. Place almond butter in a dipping bowl for a communal setting.

Caprese Skewers

Ingredients:

- Cherry tomatoes

- Fresh mozzarella balls

- Basil leaves

- Balsamic glaze for drizzling

Preparation Time: 10 minutes

Serving Time: 5 minutes

Nutritional Info: Protein, vitamins, and antioxidants.

Instructions:

- Thread a cherry tomato, a mozzarella ball, and a basil leaf onto small skewers.

- Arrange on a serving platter.

- Drizzle with balsamic glaze before serving.

Serving Methods:

1. Serve on a platter for an elegant presentation.

2. Create a DIY station with components for guests to assemble their skewers.

Edamame and Sea Salt Pods

Ingredients:

- 1 cup edamame pods

- Sea salt for sprinkling

Preparation Time: 5 minutes

Cooking Time: 5 minutes

Serving Time: 5 minutes

Nutritional Info: Plant-based protein and minerals.

Instructions:

- Boil edamame pods in salted water for 5 minutes.

- Drain and sprinkle with sea salt.

- Serve in a bowl for easy snacking.

Serving Methods:

1. Place in a bowl for an individual serving.

2. Serve in a larger bowl for sharing.

Whole Grain Crackers with Tuna Salad

Ingredients:

- Whole grain crackers

- 1 can (5 oz.) tuna, drained

- 1/4 cup Greek yogurt

- 1 tablespoon Dijon mustard

- Celery, finely chopped

- Salt and pepper to taste

Preparation Time: 10 minutes

Serving Time: 5 minutes

Nutritional Info: Protein, whole grains, and omega-3s.

Instructions:

- In a bowl, mix tuna, Greek yogurt, Dijon mustard, celery, salt, and pepper.

- Spoon the tuna salad onto whole grain crackers.

- Arrange on a serving plate.

Serving Methods:

1. Place individual crackers on a plate for easy consumption.

2. Set up a build-your-own station with separate bowls for components.

Spinach and Artichoke Dip with Veggie Sticks

Ingredients:

- 2 cups fresh spinach, chopped

- 1 can (14 oz.) artichoke hearts, drained and chopped

- 1 cup Greek yogurt

- 1/2 cup grated Parmesan cheese

- 1 clove garlic, minced

- Assorted veggie sticks (carrots, celery, bell peppers)

Preparation Time: 15 minutes

Serving Time: 5 minutes

Nutritional Info: Fiber, vitamins, and probiotics.

Instructions:

- In a bowl, combine chopped spinach, artichoke hearts, Greek yogurt, Parmesan cheese, and minced garlic.

- Mix until well combined.

- Serve with assorted veggie sticks for dipping.

Serving Methods:

1. Place dip in a bowl surrounded by veggie sticks.

2. Portion into individual containers for personal snacking.

Roasted Red Pepper Hummus with Pita Chips

Ingredients:

- 1 can (15 oz.) chickpeas, drained and rinsed

- 1/2 cup roasted red peppers

- 1/4 cup tahini

- 2 tablespoons lemon juice

- 2 cloves garlic, minced

- Pita chips for dipping

Preparation Time: 10 minutes

Serving Time: 5 minutes

Nutritional Info: Plant-based protein, fiber, and vitamins.

Instructions:

- In a food processor, blend chickpeas, roasted red peppers, tahini, lemon juice, and minced garlic until smooth.

- Serve in a bowl with pita chips for dipping.

Serving Methods:

1. Place in the center of a snack table with a bowl of pita chips.

2. Portion into smaller bowls for individual servings.

Sweet Potato and Chickpea Patties

Ingredients:

- 1 cup cooked sweet potatoes, mashed

- 1 can (15 oz.) chickpeas, drained and mashed

- 2 tablespoons almond flour

- 1 teaspoon cumin

- 1/2 teaspoon paprika

- Salt and pepper to taste

- Greek yogurt sauce for dipping

Preparation Time: 15 minutes

Cooking Time: 20 minutes

Serving Time: 5 minutes

Nutritional Info: Fiber, plant-based protein, and vitamins.

Instructions:

- In a bowl, mix mashed sweet potatoes, mashed chickpeas, almond flour, cumin, paprika, salt, and pepper.

- Form into small patties.

- Cook on a skillet until golden brown on both sides.

- Serve with a side of Greek yogurt sauce.

Serving Methods:

1. Arrange on a platter for sharing.

2. Serve individually as a quick grab-and-go snack.

Cinnamon Apple Chips

Ingredients:

- 2 apples, thinly sliced

- 1 tablespoon cinnamon

- 1 tablespoon coconut sugar (optional)

- Nut butter for dipping

Preparation Time: 10 minutes

Baking Time: 2-3 hours

Serving Time: 5 minutes

Nutritional Info: *Fiber, natural sugars, and healthy fats*

Instructions:

- Preheat the oven to 200°F (95°C).

- Toss apple slices in cinnamon and coconut sugar.

- Arrange on a baking sheet.

- Bake until crisp.

- Serve with a side of nut butter for dipping.

Serving Methods:

1. Place in a bowl for an individual serving.

2. Arrange on a serving tray for a shared snack.

Quinoa and Veggie Stuffed Mushrooms

Ingredients:

- 1 cup cooked quinoa

- 1/2 cup bell peppers, finely diced

- 1/4 cup red onion, finely chopped

- 1/4 cup feta cheese, crumbled

- Mushrooms, cleaned and stems removed

- Olive oil for drizzling

- Fresh parsley for garnish

Preparation Time: 15 minutes

Baking Time: 20 minutes

Serving Time: 5 minutes

Nutritional Info: Protein, fiber, and vitamins.

Instructions:

- Preheat the oven to 375°F (190°C).

- In a bowl, mix cooked quinoa, diced bell peppers, red onion, and feta cheese.

- Stuff mushrooms with the quinoa mixture.

- Drizzle with olive oil and bake until mushrooms are tender.

- Garnish with fresh parsley before serving.

Serving Methods:

1. Arrange on a platter for an elegant presentation.

2. Serve individually as a portioned snack.

Chia Seed Pudding with Berries

Ingredients:

- 1/4 cup chia seeds

- 1 cup almond milk

- 1 tablespoon maple syrup

- Mixed berries for topping

- Nuts for garnish

Preparation Time: 5 minutes (plus chilling time)

Serving Time: 5 minutes

Nutritional Info: Omega-3s, fiber, and antioxidants.

Instructions:

- Mix chia seeds, almond milk, and maple syrup in a jar.

- Refrigerate for a few hours or overnight until it forms a pudding-like consistency.

- Layer with mixed berries.

- Garnish with nuts before serving.

Serving Methods:

1. Serve in individual jars.

2. Create a parfait by layering in a glass.

Avocado and Black Bean Salsa

Ingredients:

- 1 ripe avocado, diced

- 1 can (15 oz.) black beans, drained and rinsed

- 1/2 cup corn kernels

- 1/4 cup red onion, finely chopped

- Lime juice for dressing

- Fresh cilantro for garnish

- Whole grain tortilla chips for dipping

Preparation Time: 10 minutes

Serving Time: 5 minutes

Nutritional Info: Healthy fats, fiber, and vitamins.

Instructions:

- In a bowl, combine diced avocado, black beans, corn, and red onion.

- Drizzle with lime juice and toss gently.

- Garnish with fresh cilantro.

- Serve with whole grain tortilla chips.

Serving Methods:

1. Present in a bowl for individual servings.

2. Set up a snack station with separate bowls for components.

Cucumber Roll-Ups with Smoked Salmon

Ingredients:

- 1 cucumber, thinly sliced lengthwise

- 4 oz. smoked salmon

- Cream cheese

- Dill for garnish

Preparation Time: 15 minutes

Serving Time: 5 minutes

Nutritional Info: Omega-3s, protein, and vitamins.

Instructions:

- Spread a thin layer of cream cheese on each cucumber slice.

- Place a piece of smoked salmon on top.

- Roll up and secure with a toothpick.

- Garnish with fresh dill.

Serving Methods:

1. Arrange on a plate for an elegant presentation.

2. Serve on a platter for a party or gathering.

Pumpkin Seed and Dried Cherry Mix

Ingredients:

- 1 cup pumpkin seeds, toasted

- 1/2 cup dried cherries

- 1/4 cup dark chocolate chips

- 1/4 teaspoon sea salt

Preparation Time: 5 minutes

Serving Time: 5 minutes

Nutritional Info: Protein, antioxidants, and healthy fats.

Instructions:

- In a bowl, mix pumpkin seeds, dried cherries, dark chocolate chips, and sea salt.

- Toss until well combined.

- Portion into small snack-sized bags.

- Serve as needed.

Serving Methods:

1. Hand out individual bags for a quick grab-and-go snack.

2. Display on a serving tray for a shared snacking experience.

Carrot and Hummus Dippers

Ingredients:

- Carrot sticks

- Hummus

- Sesame seeds for garnish

Preparation Time: 10 minutes

Serving Time: 5 minutes

Nutritional Info: Fiber, plant-based protein, and vitamins.

Instructions:

- Arrange carrot sticks on a plate.

- Serve with a side of hummus.

- Sprinkle sesame seeds for added crunch.

Serving Methods:

1. Place on a platter for a party.

2. Portion into individual containers for personal snacking.

Rice Cake with Almond Butter and Banana Slices

Ingredients:

- Rice cakes
- Almond butter
- Banana, sliced
- Chia seeds for topping

Preparation Time: 5 minutes

Serving Time: 5 minutes

Nutritional Info: Fiber, healthy fats, and natural sugars.

Instructions:

- Spread almond butter on rice cakes.
- Top with banana slices.
- Sprinkle chia seeds for extra nutrition.
- Serve on a plate.

Serving Methods:

1. Arrange on a plate for an individual snack.

2. Set up a topping station for customization in a group setting.

Blueberry and Almond Oat Bars

Ingredients:

- 2 cups rolled oats

- 1 cup almond butter

- 1/2 cup honey

- 1/2 cup dried blueberries

- 1/4 cup almonds, chopped

- Vanilla extract

- Pinch of salt

Preparation Time: 15 minutes

Baking Time: 15 minutes

Serving Time: 5 minutes

Nutritional Info: Fiber, protein, and antioxidants.

Instructions:

- Mix rolled oats, almond butter, honey, dried blueberries, chopped almonds, vanilla extract, and a pinch of salt in a bowl.

- Press the mixture into a lined baking dish.

- Bake until set and golden brown.

- Allow to cool, then cut into bars.

- Serve on a plate or in snack bags.

Serving Methods:

1. Present on a plate for individual servings.

2. Pack in snack-sized bags for on-the-go convenience.

CHAPTER TEN

BEVERAGES RECIPES

Minty Blueberry Lemonade

Ingredients:

- 1 cup blueberries (fresh or frozen)

- 2 tablespoons fresh mint leaves

- 2 tablespoons honey

- 1 lemon, juiced

- 4 cups cold water

- Ice cubes

Preparation Time: 10 minutes

Serving Time: 5 minutes

Nutritional Info: Antioxidants, vitamin C, and hydration.

Instructions:

- In a blender, combine blueberries, mint leaves, honey, and lemon juice.

- Blend until smooth.

- Strain the mixture into a pitcher.

- Add cold water and stir.

- Serve over ice.

Serving Methods:

1. Pour into individual glasses.

2. Present in a pitcher for sharing.

Turmeric Mango Smoothie

Ingredients:

- 1 cup mango chunks (fresh or frozen)

- 1/2 teaspoon turmeric powder

- 1/2 teaspoon ginger powder

- 1 cup coconut milk

- 1 tablespoon chia seeds

- Ice cubes

Preparation Time: 5 minutes

Serving Time: 5 minutes

Nutritional Info: Anti-inflammatory properties, fiber, and omega-3s.

Instructions:

- Blend mango chunks, turmeric powder, ginger powder, coconut milk, and chia seeds until smooth.

- Add ice cubes and blend again.

- Pour into a glass and enjoy.

Serving Methods:

1. Serve in a tall glass.

2. Pour into a travel cup for on-the-go convenience.

Cherry Almond Protein Shake

Ingredients:

- 1 cup cherries (fresh or frozen)

- 1 tablespoon almond butter

- 1/2 cup Greek yogurt

- 1 cup almond milk

- 1 teaspoon honey (optional)

- Ice cubes

Preparation Time: 7 minutes

Serving Time: 5 minutes

Nutritional Info: Protein, healthy fats, and vitamins.

Instructions:

- Blend cherries, almond butter, Greek yogurt, almond milk, and honey until creamy.

- Add ice cubes and blend for a cool texture.

- Pour into a glass and serve.

Serving Methods:

1. Garnish with a cherry on top for individual servings.

2. Prepare in a blender bottle for a portable drink.

Cucumber Basil Sparkling Water

Ingredients:

- 1 cucumber, sliced

- 1/4 cup fresh basil leaves

- 1 tablespoon lime juice

- 2 cups sparkling water

- Ice cubes

Preparation Time: 5 minutes

Serving Time: 5 minutes

Nutritional Info: Hydration, antioxidants, and vitamins.

Instructions:

- In a pitcher, combine cucumber slices, basil leaves, and lime juice.

- Add sparkling water and stir gently.

- Refrigerate for at least 1 hour.

- Serve over ice.

Serving Methods:

1. Use a ladle to serve in individual glasses.

2. Present in a large jug for a group gathering.

Pineapple Ginger Iced Tea

Ingredients:

- 2 black tea bags

- 1 cup pineapple chunks

- 1 tablespoon fresh ginger, grated

- 2 tablespoons honey

- 4 cups cold water

- Ice cubes

Preparation Time: 10 minutes

Serving Time: 5 minutes

Nutritional Info: Antioxidants, digestive benefits, and hydration.

Instructions:

- Brew black tea bags in hot water, then allow it to cool.

- In a blender, combine pineapple chunks, grated ginger, and honey. Blend until smooth.

- Strain the pineapple mixture into the brewed tea.

- Stir well and refrigerate.

- Serve over ice.

Serving Methods:

1. Pour into individual glasses.

2. Present in a large pitcher with pineapple and ginger garnish.

Beetroot Berry Detox Juice

Ingredients:

- 1 medium-sized beetroot, peeled and chopped

- 1 cup mixed berries (strawberries, blueberries, raspberries)

- 1/2 cucumber, peeled and sliced

- 1 tablespoon lemon juice

- 2 cups cold water

- Ice cubes

Preparation Time: 10 minutes

Serving Time: 5 minutes

Nutritional Info: Detoxifying, vitamins, and hydration.

Instructions:

- In a blender, combine beetroot, mixed berries, cucumber, lemon juice, and cold water.

- Blend until smooth.

- Strain the mixture into a pitcher.

- Refrigerate for at least 1 hour.

- Serve over ice.

Serving Methods:

1. Use a ladle to pour into individual glasses.

2. Present in a glass pitcher for a colorful display.

Coconut Watermelon Refresher

Ingredients:

- 2 cups fresh watermelon, cubed

- 1 cup coconut water

- 1 tablespoon lime juice

- 1 tablespoon mint leaves, chopped

- Ice cubes

Preparation Time: 8 minutes

Serving Time: 5 minutes

Nutritional Info: Hydration, vitamins, and electrolytes.

Instructions:

- In a blender, combine watermelon, coconut water, lime juice, and mint leaves.

- Blend until smooth.

- Strain the mixture into a pitcher.

- Refrigerate for at least 30 minutes.

- Serve over ice.

Serving Methods:

1. Pour into individual glasses.

2. Serve in coconut halves for a tropical presentation.

Matcha Avocado Smoothie

Ingredients:

- 1 teaspoon matcha powder

- 1/2 avocado, peeled and pitted

- 1 banana

- 1 cup almond milk

- 1 teaspoon honey (optional)

- Ice cubes

Preparation Time: 7 minutes

Serving Time: 5 minutes

Nutritional Info: Antioxidants, healthy fats, and vitamins.

Instructions:

- Blend matcha powder, avocado, banana, almond milk, and honey until creamy.

- Add ice cubes and blend for a refreshing texture.

- Pour into a glass and serve.

Serving Methods:

1. Garnish with a slice of avocado for an individual serving.

2. Prepare in a travel cup for a nutrient-rich snack on the go.

Raspberry Hibiscus Iced Tea

Ingredients:

- 2 hibiscus tea bags

- 1 cup fresh raspberries

- 2 tablespoons agave syrup

- 4 cups cold water

- Ice cubes

Preparation Time: 10 minutes

Serving Time: 5 minutes

Nutritional Info: Antioxidants, vitamins, and hydration.

Instructions:

- Brew hibiscus tea bags in hot water and allow it to cool.

- In a blender, combine raspberries and agave syrup. Blend until smooth.

- Strain the raspberry mixture into the brewed tea.

- Stir well and refrigerate.

- Serve over ice.

Serving Methods:

1. Pour into individual glasses.

2. Present in a large pitcher with whole raspberries for decoration.

Peach Ginger Kombucha Cooler

Ingredients:

- 1 peach, sliced

- 1 tablespoon fresh ginger, grated

- 2 cups peach-flavored kombucha

- 1 tablespoon honey (optional)

- Ice cubes

Preparation Time: 8 minutes

Serving Time: 5 minutes

Nutritional Info: Probiotics, digestion support, and hydration.

Instructions:

- In a pitcher, combine sliced peach, grated ginger, and peach-flavored kombucha.

- Add honey if additional sweetness is desired.

- Stir gently and refrigerate for at least 1 hour.

- Serve over ice.

Serving Methods:

1. Use a ladle to pour into individual glasses.

2. Present in a glass dispenser with peach and ginger slices.

Citrus Mint Infused Water

Ingredients:

- 1 lemon, sliced

- 1 lime, sliced

- 1 orange, sliced

- Fresh mint leaves

- 4 cups cold water

- Ice cubes

Preparation Time: 10 minutes

Serving Time: 5 minutes

Nutritional Info: Hydration, vitamin C, and antioxidants.

Instructions:

- Combine lemon, lime, orange slices, and mint leaves in a pitcher.

- Add cold water and stir.

- Refrigerate for at least 1 hour.

- Serve over ice.

Serving Methods:

1. Pour into individual glasses.

2. Present in a large pitcher for sharing.

Cranberry Apple Cinnamon Tea

Ingredients:

- 2 black tea bags

- 1 cup cranberry juice (unsweetened)

- 1 apple, sliced

- 1 cinnamon stick

- 4 cups hot water

- Honey to taste (optional)

Preparation Time: 8 minutes

Serving Time: 5 minutes

Nutritional Info: Antioxidants, hydration, and vitamins.

Instructions:

- Brew black tea bags in hot water.

- In a pitcher, combine cranberry juice, apple slices, and a cinnamon stick.

- Pour in the brewed tea.

- Sweeten with honey if desired.

- Allow it to cool, then refrigerate.

- Serve over ice.

Serving Methods:

1. Pour into individual cups.

2. Present in a teapot for a cozy gathering.

Pineapple Basil Smoothie

Ingredients:

- 1 cup pineapple chunks

- 1/2 cup fresh basil leaves

- 1/2 cup Greek yogurt

- 1 cup coconut water

- Ice cubes

Preparation Time: 7 minutes

Serving Time: 5 minutes

Nutritional Info: Digestive support, hydration, and vitamins.

Instructions:

- Blend pineapple chunks, basil leaves, Greek yogurt, and coconut water until smooth.

- Add ice cubes and blend for a refreshing texture.

- Pour into glasses and serve.

Serving Methods:

1. Garnish with a basil leaf for individual servings.

2. Prepare in a large jug for a brunch setting.

Mango Mint Lassi

Ingredients:

- 1 cup ripe mango, diced

- 1/2 cup plain yogurt

- Fresh mint leaves

- 1 tablespoon honey

- 1 cup cold water

- Ice cubes

Preparation Time: 6 minutes

Serving Time: 5 minutes

Nutritional Info: Probiotics, hydration, and vitamins.

Instructions:

- In a blender, combine diced mango, plain yogurt, mint leaves, honey, and cold water.

- Blend until smooth.

- Add ice cubes and blend again.

- Pour into glasses and serve.

Serving Methods:

1. Garnish with a mint sprig for individual servings.

2. Present in small mason jars for a rustic touch.

Blueberry Almond Milkshake

Ingredients:

- 1 cup blueberries (fresh or frozen)

- 1/2 cup almond milk

- 2 tablespoons almond butter

- 1 tablespoon flaxseeds

- 1 teaspoon vanilla extract

- Ice cubes

Preparation Time: 6 minutes

Serving Time: 5 minutes

Nutritional Info: Omega-3s, antioxidants, and vitamins.

Instructions:

- Blend blueberries, almond milk, almond butter, flaxseeds, and vanilla extract until creamy.

- Add ice cubes and blend for a chilled consistency.

- Pour into glasses and serve.

Serving Methods:

1. Garnish with a few blueberries for individual servings.

2. Present in a tall glass for an elegant look.

Carrot Ginger Turmeric Elixir

Ingredients:

- 1 cup carrot juice

- 1 teaspoon fresh ginger, grated

- 1/2 teaspoon turmeric powder

- 1 tablespoon lemon juice

- 2 cups cold water

- Ice cubes

Preparation Time: 8 minutes

Serving Time: 5 minutes

Nutritional Info: Anti-inflammatory properties, hydration, and vitamins.

Instructions:

- In a pitcher, combine carrot juice, grated ginger, turmeric powder, lemon juice, and cold water.

- Stir well and refrigerate for at least 1 hour.

- Serve over ice.

Serving Methods:

1. Pour into individual glasses.

2. Present in a glass dispenser for a health-conscious gathering.

Strawberry Basil Lemonade

Ingredients:

- 1 cup strawberries, hulled

- Fresh basil leaves

- 1/4 cup honey

- 1 lemon, juiced

- 4 cups cold water

- Ice cubes

Preparation Time: 10 minutes

Serving Time: 5 minutes

Nutritional Info: Hydration, vitamin C, and antioxidants.

Instructions:

- Blend strawberries, basil leaves, honey, and lemon juice until smooth.

- Strain the mixture into a pitcher.

- Add cold water and stir.

- Refrigerate for at least 1 hour.

- Serve over ice.

Serving Methods:

1. Pour into individual glasses.

2. Present in a clear pitcher for a vibrant display.

Cherry Vanilla Chia Seed Pudding Smoothie

Ingredients:

- 1/2 cup cherries (pitted)

- 1/2 cup almond milk

- 1 tablespoon chia seeds

- 1/2 teaspoon vanilla extract

- 1 tablespoon protein powder (optional)

- Ice cubes

Preparation Time: 7 minutes

Serving Time: 5 minutes

Nutritional Info: Omega-3s, protein, and vitamins.

Instructions:

- Blend cherries, almond milk, chia seeds, vanilla extract, and protein powder until smooth.

- Add ice cubes and blend for a thick texture.

- Pour into glasses and serve.

Serving Methods:

1. Garnish with a cherry for individual servings.

2. Prepare in a travel cup for a nutrient-packed snack.

Melon Mint Refresher

Ingredients:

- 2 cups mixed melon balls (cantaloupe, honeydew, watermelon)

- Fresh mint leaves

- 1 tablespoon lime juice

- 2 cups coconut water

- Ice cubes

Preparation Time: 8 minutes

Serving Time: 5 minutes

Nutritional Info: Hydration, vitamins, and antioxidants

Instructions:

- In a pitcher, combine melon balls, mint leaves, lime juice, and coconut water.

- Stir gently and refrigerate for at least 1 hour.

- Serve over ice.

Serving Methods:

- Use a ladle to serve in individual glasses.

- Present in a clear bowl for a visually appealing centerpiece.

Hazelnut Mocha Protein Shake

Ingredients:

- 1 cup cold brew coffee
- 1/2 cup hazelnut milk
- 1 tablespoon cocoa powder
- 1 tablespoon hazelnut butter
- 1 scoop chocolate protein powder
- Ice cubes

Preparation Time: 7 minutes

Serving Time: 5 minutes

Nutritional Info: Protein, antioxidants, and healthy fats.

Instructions:

- In a blender, combine cold brew coffee, hazelnut milk, cocoa powder, hazelnut butter, and chocolate protein powder.
- Blend until smooth.
- Add ice cubes and blend for a creamy texture.
- Pour into glasses and serve.

Serving Methods:

1. Garnish with a sprinkle of cocoa powder for individual servings.

2. Prepare in a shaker bottle for a convenient on-the-go option.

CHAPTER ELEVEN

DESSERT RECIPES

Berry Bliss Parfait

Ingredients:

- 1 cup mixed berries (strawberries, blueberries, raspberries)

- 1 cup low-fat Greek yogurt

- 2 tablespoons honey

- 1/4 cup granola

Preparation Time: 10 minutes

Cooking Time: No cooking required

Serving Time: 15 minutes

Nutritional Info:

- Calories: 200

- Protein: 10g

- Fiber: 5g

- Sugar: 15g

Instructions:

- In a glass, layer mixed berries at the bottom.

- Add a spoonful of Greek yogurt on top.

- Drizzle with honey and sprinkle granola.

- Repeat the layers.

- Serve chilled.

Serving Methods:

1. Serve in individual glasses for an elegant presentation.

2. Create a larger serving in a trifle bowl for a family-style dessert.

Avocado Chocolate Mousse

Ingredients:

- 2 ripe avocados

- 1/4 cup unsweetened cocoa powder

- 1/4 cup honey

- 1 teaspoon vanilla extract

- Pinch of salt

Preparation Time: 15 minutes

Cooking Time: No cooking required

Serving Time: 30 minutes

Nutritional Info:

- Calories: 180

- Protein: 3g

- Healthy Fats: 15g

- Sugar: 10g

Instructions:

- In a blender, combine avocados, cocoa powder, honey, vanilla extract, and a pinch of salt.

- Blend until smooth and creamy.

- Refrigerate for 15 minutes before serving.

- Garnish with fresh berries or mint.

Serving Methods:

1. Spoon the mousse into individual bowls for a personalized touch.

2. Serve with a dollop of whipped cream for added indulgence.

Apple Walnut Crisp

Ingredients:

- 4 apples, peeled and sliced

- 1 cup rolled oats

- 1/2 cup chopped walnuts

- 1/4 cup maple syrup

- 1 teaspoon cinnamon

Preparation Time: 20 minutes

Cooking Time: 30 minutes

Serving Time: 45 minutes

Nutritional Info:

- Calories: 250

- Fiber: 7g

- Protein: 5g

- Sugar: 20g

Instructions:

- Preheat oven to 350°F (175°C).

- In a bowl, toss sliced apples with maple syrup and cinnamon.

- In a separate bowl, combine rolled oats and chopped walnuts.

- In a baking dish, layer the apple mixture and top with the oat and walnut mixture.

- Bake for 30 minutes or until the top is golden brown.

- Serve warm.

Serving Methods:

1. Top with a scoop of vanilla frozen yogurt.

2. Drizzle with caramel sauce for an extra decadent treat.

Banana Almond Bites

Ingredients:

- 2 ripe bananas, mashed

- 1/2 cup almond flour

- 1/4 cup shredded coconut

- 1/4 cup dark chocolate chips

- 1 teaspoon vanilla extract

Preparation Time: 15 minutes

Cooking Time: 15 minutes

Serving Time: 30 minutes

Nutritional Info:

- Calories: 180

- Protein: 4g

- Healthy Fats: 10g

- Sugar: 10g

Instructions:

- Preheat oven to 350°F (175°C).

- In a bowl, combine mashed bananas, almond flour, shredded coconut, dark chocolate chips, and vanilla extract.

- Mix until well combined.

- Drop spoonfuls onto a baking sheet lined with parchment paper.

- Bake for 15 minutes or until golden brown.

- Allow to cool before serving.

Serving Methods:

1. Arrange on a dessert platter for a casual gathering.

2. Serve with a dusting of powdered sugar for a touch of elegance.

Chia Seed Pudding with Mango

Ingredients:

- 1/4 cup chia seeds

- 1 cup almond milk

- 1 tablespoon honey

- 1/2 teaspoon vanilla extract

- 1 ripe mango, diced

Preparation Time: 5 minutes (plus overnight chilling)

Cooking Time: No cooking required

Serving Time: 10 minutes

Nutritional Info:

- Calories: 180

- Fiber: 8g

- Protein: 4g

- Sugar: 15g

Instructions:

- In a bowl, mix chia seeds, almond milk, honey, and vanilla extract.

- Stir well and refrigerate overnight or for at least 4 hours.

- Before serving, stir the pudding to ensure a smooth consistency.

- Top with diced mango.

Serving Methods:

1. Serve in small jars for a stylish individual presentation.

2. Layer with granola for added texture and flavor.

Lemon Blueberry Frozen Yogurt

Ingredients:

- 2 cups frozen blueberries

- 1 cup Greek yogurt

- 1/4 cup honey

- Zest and juice of 1 lemon

Preparation Time: 10 minutes

Cooking Time: No cooking required

Serving Time: 20 minutes

Nutritional Info:

- Calories: 150

- Protein: 8g

- Fiber: 3g

- Sugar: 15g

Instructions:

- In a blender, combine frozen blueberries, Greek yogurt, honey, lemon zest, and lemon juice.

- Blend until smooth.

- Scoop into serving bowls or cones.

- Serve immediately.

Serving Methods:

1. Top with fresh mint leaves for a burst of freshness.

2. Layer with additional fresh berries for a colorful presentation.

Cinnamon Baked Pears

Ingredients:

- 4 ripe pears, halved and cored

- 2 tablespoons melted butter

- 2 tablespoons honey

- 1 teaspoon cinnamon

- 1/4 cup chopped pecans

Preparation Time: 10 minutes

Cooking Time: 25 minutes

Serving Time: 35 minutes

Nutritional Info:

- Calories: 200

- Fiber: 6g

- Healthy Fats: 10g

- Sugar: 15g

Instructions:

1. Preheat oven to 375°F (190°C).

2. Place pear halves on a baking sheet.

3. In a bowl, mix melted butter, honey, and cinnamon.

4. Brush the mixture over the pears.

5. Bake for 25 minutes or until pears are tender.

6. Sprinkle with chopped pecans before serving.

Serving Methods:

- Serve with a scoop of vanilla ice cream for an indulgent treat.

- Drizzle with caramel sauce for added sweetness.

Almond Joy Energy Bites

Ingredients:

- 1 cup rolled oats

- 1/2 cup almond butter

- 1/4 cup honey

- 1/4 cup shredded coconut

- 1/4 cup dark chocolate chips

Preparation Time: 15 minutes

Cooking Time: No cooking required

Serving Time: 30 minutes

Nutritional Info:

- Calories: 160

- Protein: 5g

- Healthy Fats: 8g

- Sugar: 8g

Instructions:

- In a bowl, combine rolled oats, almond butter, honey, shredded coconut, and dark chocolate chips.

- Mix until well combined.

- Roll into bite-sized balls.

- Refrigerate for 15 minutes before serving.

Serving Methods:

1. Arrange on a dessert platter for casual gatherings.

2. Serve in mini cupcake liners for a convenient and portable dessert.

Peach Sorbet

Ingredients:

- 4 ripe peaches, peeled and sliced

- 1/4 cup honey

- Juice of 1 lime

- 1/2 cup coconut water

Preparation Time: 10 minutes

Cooking Time: No cooking required

Serving Time: 25 minutes

Nutritional Info:

- Calories: 120

- Fiber: 3g

- Vitamin C: 10mg

- Sugar: 15g

Instructions:

1. In a blender, combine sliced peaches, honey, lime juice, and coconut water.

2. Blend until smooth.

3. Pour into a shallow dish and freeze for 4 hours, stirring every hour.

4. Scoop and serve.

Serving Methods:

- Garnish with mint leaves for a refreshing touch.

- Serve in chilled bowls for a cool presentation.

Pumpkin Spice Chia Pudding

Ingredients:

- 1/4 cup chia seeds

- 1 cup almond milk

- 1/4 cup pumpkin puree

- 2 tablespoons maple syrup

- 1/2 teaspoon pumpkin spice

Preparation Time: 10 minutes (plus chilling time)

Cooking Time: No cooking required

Serving Time: 15 minutes

Nutritional Info:

- Calories: 180

- Fiber: 7g

- Protein: 5g

- Sugar: 10g

Instructions:

- In a bowl, mix chia seeds, almond milk, pumpkin puree, maple syrup, and pumpkin spice.

- Stir well and refrigerate for at least 4 hours or overnight.

- Stir before serving.

- Top with a sprinkle of additional pumpkin spice.

Serving Methods:

1. Layer with crushed graham crackers for a pumpkin pie-inspired dessert.

2. Serve in small mason jars for a visually appealing individual presentation.

Recipe 1: Dark Chocolate Avocado Mousse

Ingredients:

- 2 ripe avocados

- 1/4 cup unsweetened dark cocoa powder

- 1/4 cup maple syrup

- 1 teaspoon vanilla extract

- Pinch of sea salt

Preparation Time: 15 minutes

Cooking Time: No cooking required

Serving Time: 30 minutes

Nutritional Info:

- Calories: 200

- Protein: 4g

- Healthy Fats: 15g

- Sugar: 10g

Instructions:

- In a blender, combine avocados, cocoa powder, maple syrup, vanilla extract, and sea salt.

- Blend until silky smooth.

- Refrigerate for at least 15 minutes before serving.

- Garnish with shaved dark chocolate or fresh berries.

Serving Methods:

1. Spoon into individual ramekins for an elegant presentation.

2. Serve with a dollop of coconut whipped cream for added richness.

Almond and Berry Quinoa Parfait

Ingredients:

- 1 cup cooked quinoa, cooled

- 1/2 cup almond milk

- 1 tablespoon honey

- 1/2 cup mixed berries (strawberries, blueberries, raspberries)

- 2 tablespoons sliced almonds

Preparation Time: 20 minutes

Cooking Time: 15 minutes (for quinoa)

Serving Time: 30 minutes

Nutritional Info:

- Calories: 220

- Protein: 6g

- Fiber: 5g

- Sugar: 10g

Instructions:

1. In a bowl, mix quinoa with almond milk and honey.

2. Layer the quinoa mixture with mixed berries in serving glasses.

3. Repeat the layers.

4. Top with sliced almonds.

5. Chill before serving.

Serving Methods:

- Present in tall glasses for a visually appealing dessert.

- Garnish with a mint sprig for a burst of color.

Pumpkin Spice Chia Pudding

Ingredients:

- 1/4 cup chia seeds

- 1 cup unsweetened almond milk

- 1/4 cup canned pumpkin puree

- 1 tablespoon maple syrup

- 1/2 teaspoon pumpkin spice blend

Preparation Time: 10 minutes (plus chilling time)

Cooking Time: No cooking required

Serving Time: 20 minutes

Nutritional Info:

- Calories: 180

- Fiber: 8g

- Protein: 4g

- Sugar: 6g

Instructions:

- In a bowl, whisk together chia seeds, almond milk, pumpkin puree, maple syrup, and pumpkin spice.

- Refrigerate for at least 2 hours or overnight.

- Stir before serving.

- Garnish with a sprinkle of additional pumpkin spice.

Serving Methods:

1. Serve in small jars for a delightful individual dessert.

2. Top with a dollop of coconut yogurt for added creaminess.

Mango Coconut Rice Pudding

Ingredients:

- 1/2 cup Arborio rice

- 2 cups coconut milk

- 1/4 cup honey

- 1 ripe mango, diced

- 2 tablespoons shredded coconut

Preparation Time: 10 minutes

Cooking Time: 30 minutes

Serving Time: 45 minutes

Nutritional Info:

- Calories: 250

- Protein: 3g

- Healthy Fats: 10g

- Sugar: 15g

Instructions:

- In a saucepan, combine rice and coconut milk.

- Simmer over low heat, stirring frequently, until rice is tender.

- Stir in honey and cook for an additional 5 minutes.

- Allow the pudding to cool before adding diced mango and shredded coconut.

- Serve chilled.

Serving Methods:

1. Present in coconut shells for a tropical flair.

2. Drizzle with a passion fruit coulis for an exotic touch.

Blueberry Lemon Yogurt Parfait

Ingredients:

- 1 cup Greek yogurt

- 1 cup fresh blueberries

- 2 tablespoons honey

- Zest of 1 lemon

- 1/4 cup granola

Preparation Time: 15 minutes

Cooking Time: No cooking required

Serving Time: 30 minutes

Nutritional Info:

- Calories: 220

- Protein: 10g

- Fiber: 3g

- Sugar: 15g

Instructions:

1. In a glass, layer Greek yogurt with fresh blueberries.

2. Drizzle honey over the layers and sprinkle lemon zest.

3. Repeat the layers.

4. Top with granola just before serving.

Serving Methods:

- Serve in transparent bowls to showcase the vibrant layers.

- Garnish with a lemon twist for an added visual element.

Raspberry Coconut Chia Popsicles

Ingredients:

- 1/4 cup chia seeds

- 1 cup coconut milk

- 1 cup fresh raspberries

- 2 tablespoons agave syrup

- Popsicle molds

Preparation Time: 10 minutes (plus freezing time)

Cooking Time: No cooking required

Serving Time: 4 hours (freezing time)

Nutritional Info:

- Calories: 150

- Fiber: 6g

- Protein: 3g

- Sugar: 8g

Instructions:

- In a blender, mix chia seeds with coconut milk and
  agave syrup.

- Let the mixture sit for 15 minutes to allow chia seeds to gel.

- Fill popsicle molds halfway with the chia mixture.

- Add a layer of fresh raspberries.

- Top with the remaining chia mixture.

- Freeze for at least 4 hours.

Serving Methods:

1. Serve as a refreshing dessert on a hot day.

2. Dip the popsicles in shredded coconut for an extra crunch.

Apple Cinnamon Oat Bars

Ingredients:

- 2 cups rolled oats

- 1 cup unsweetened applesauce

- 1/4 cup almond butter

- 1/4 cup maple syrup

- 1 teaspoon cinnamon

Preparation Time: 15 minutes

Cooking Time: 25 minutes

Serving Time: 40 minutes

Nutritional Info:

- Calories: 180

- Fiber: 5g

- Protein: 4g

- Sugar: 8g

Instructions:

1. Preheat oven to 350°F (175°C).

2. In a bowl, combine rolled oats, applesauce, almond butter, maple syrup, and cinnamon.

3. Press the mixture into a baking dish.

4. Bake for 25 minutes or until golden brown.

5. Allow to cool before cutting into bars.

Serving Methods:

1. Serve as handheld bars for convenience.

2. Pair with a scoop of vanilla yogurt for added creaminess.

Peach Basil Sorbet

Ingredients:

- 2 cups frozen peach slices

- 1/4 cup fresh basil leaves

- 1/4 cup honey

- Juice of 1 lime

Preparation Time: 10 minutes

Cooking Time: No cooking required

Serving Time: 20 minutes

Nutritional Info:

- Calories: 120

- Fiber: 3g

- Protein: 1g

- Sugar: 15g

Instructions:

- In a blender, combine frozen peach slices, fresh basil, honey, and lime juice.

- Blend until smooth.

- Transfer to a shallow dish and freeze for 15 minutes.

- Scoop and serve.

Serving Methods:

1. Garnish with fresh basil leaves for an herbal touch.

2. Serve in chilled bowls for a refreshing dessert experience.

Chocolate Covered Banana Bites

Ingredients:

- 2 bananas, peeled and sliced

- 1/2 cup dark chocolate chips, melted

- 1/4 cup chopped nuts (almonds, pistachios)

- Popsicle sticks

Preparation Time: 20 minutes

Cooking Time: 5 minutes (for melting chocolate)

Serving Time: 30 minutes

Nutritional Info:

- Calories: 160

- Protein: 3g

- Healthy Fats: 8g

- Sugar: 10g

Instructions:

- Insert popsicle sticks into banana slices.

- Dip each banana slice into melted dark chocolate.

- Sprinkle with chopped nuts.

- Place on a parchment-lined tray and freeze for 15 minutes.

- Serve chilled.

Serving Methods:

1. Arrange on a dessert platter for a party.

2. Drizzle with additional melted chocolate for extra decadence.

Lemon Ricotta Pound Cake

Ingredients:

- 1 cup almond flour

- 1/2 cup ricotta cheese

- 1/4 cup honey

- 2 tablespoons lemon juice

- Zest of 1 lemon

- 3 eggs

Preparation Time: 20 minutes

Cooking Time: 35 minutes

Serving Time: 60 minutes

Nutritional Info:

- Calories: 220

- Protein: 8g

- Healthy Fats: 15g

- Sugar: 10g

Instructions:

- Preheat oven to 350°F (175°C).

- In a bowl, mix almond flour, ricotta cheese, honey, lemon juice, lemon zest, and eggs until well combined.

- Pour the batter into a greased loaf pan.

- Bake for 35 minutes or until a toothpick comes out clean.

- Allow to cool before slicing.

Serving Methods:

1. Serve slices with a dusting of powdered sugar.

2. Pair with a scoop of lemon sorbet for a delightful contrast.

MEAL PLAN

Day 1

- ***Breakfast:*** Berry Bliss Parfait

- ***Lunch:*** Almond and Berry Quinoa Parfait

- ***Dinner:*** Pumpkin Spice Chia Pudding

Day 2

- ***Breakfast:*** Dark Chocolate Avocado Mousse

- ***Lunch:*** Mango Coconut Rice Pudding

- ***Dinner:*** Apple Cinnamon Oat Bars

Day 3

- ***Breakfast:*** Chocolate Covered Banana Bites

- ***Lunch:*** Peach Basil Sorbet

- ***Dinner:*** Lemon Ricotta Pound Cake

Day 4

- ***Breakfast:*** Banana Almond Bites

- ***Lunch:*** Chia Seed Pudding with Mango

- ***Dinner:*** Raspberry Coconut Chia Popsicles

Day 5

- *Breakfast:* Blueberry Lemon Yogurt Parfait

- *Lunch:* Cinnamon Baked Pears

- *Dinner:* Avocado Chocolate Mousse

Day 6

- *Breakfast:* Lemon Blueberry Frozen Yogurt

- *Lunch:* Apple Walnut Crisp

- *Dinner:* Mango Coconut Rice Pudding

Day 7

- *Breakfast:* Chocolate Covered Banana Bites

- *Lunch:* Raspberry Coconut Chia Popsicles

- *Dinner:* Pumpkin Spice Chia Pudding

Day 8

- *Breakfast:* Dark Chocolate Avocado Mousse

- *Lunch:* Almond and Berry Quinoa Parfait

- *Dinner:* Lemon Ricotta Pound Cake

Day 9

- *Breakfast:* Berry Bliss Parfait

- *Lunch:* Chocolate Covered Banana Bites

- *Dinner:* Cinnamon Baked Pears

Day 10

- *Breakfast:* Blueberry Lemon Yogurt Parfait

- *Lunch:* Mango Coconut Rice Pudding

- *Dinner:* Apple Cinnamon Oat Bars

Day 11

- *Breakfast:* Banana Almond Bites

- *Lunch:* Avocado Chocolate Mousse

- *Dinner:* Raspberry Coconut Chia Popsicles

Day 12

- *Breakfast:* Lemon Blueberry Frozen Yogurt

- *Lunch:* Peach Basil Sorbet

- *Dinner:* Dark Chocolate Avocado Mousse

Day 13

- *Breakfast:* Pumpkin Spice Chia Pudding

- *Lunch:* Chocolate Covered Banana Bites

- *Dinner:* Mango Coconut Rice Pudding

Day 14

- *Breakfast:* Berry Bliss Parfait

- *Lunch:* Almond and Berry Quinoa Parfait

- *Dinner:* Apple Cinnamon Oat Bars

Day 15

- *Breakfast:* Dark Chocolate Avocado Mousse

- *Lunch:* Raspberry Coconut Chia Popsicles

- *Dinner:* Lemon Ricotta Pound Cake

Day 16

- *Breakfast:* Chocolate Covered Banana Bites

- *Lunch:* Mango Coconut Rice Pudding

- *Dinner:* Pumpkin Spice Chia Pudding

Day 17

- *Breakfast:* Lemon Blueberry Frozen Yogurt

- *Lunch:* Cinnamon Baked Pears

- *Dinner:* Avocado Chocolate Mousse

Day 18

- *Breakfast:* Blueberry Lemon Yogurt Parfait

- *Lunch:* Apple Walnut Crisp

- *Dinner:* Raspberry Coconut Chia Popsicles

Day 19

- *Breakfast:* Banana Almond Bites

- *Lunch:* Peach Basil Sorbet

- *Dinner:* Mango Coconut Rice Pudding

Day 20

- *Breakfast:* Dark Chocolate Avocado Mousse

- *Lunch:* Almond and Berry Quinoa Parfait

- *Dinner:* Lemon Ricotta Pound Cake

Day 21

- *Breakfast:* Berry Bliss Parfait

- *Lunch:* Chocolate Covered Banana Bites

- *Dinner:* Cinnamon Baked Pear

CHAPTER TWELVE

EXERCISE AND NUTRITION SYNERGY

The Interplay Between Diet and Exercise

In the intricate landscape of managing Parkinson's disease, the dynamic interplay between diet and exercise emerges as a pivotal element in enhancing overall well-being. This professional discourse seeks to delve into the nuanced relationship between these two fundamental aspects of health and their profound impact on individuals navigating the challenges of Parkinson's.

Understanding Parkinson's-specific Needs

- ***Nutritional Adaptations:*** Parkinson's disease brings forth specific nutritional demands and alters exercise tolerance. As the disease progresses, the body's requirements evolve, necessitating a nuanced approach to both dietary choices and physical activity.

Fueling the Body: Pre-Exercise Nutrition

- ***Optimal Nutrient Intake:*** Before engaging in physical activity, the body requires a strategic infusion of nutrients. We explore the importance of pre-exercise nutrition, offering guidelines on meals and snacks tailored to Parkinson's patients, ensuring they embark on their fitness journeys adequately fueled.

Energizing Workouts: During Exercise Nutrition

- ***Sustaining Energy Levels:*** During exercise, maintaining optimal energy levels becomes paramount. We examine hydration and nutrition strategies designed to sustain individuals with Parkinson's throughout their physical exertion, addressing unique considerations that may arise during workout sessions.

Recovery and Nutrition Post-Exercise

- ***Prioritizing Recovery:*** Post-exercise, the body undergoes a critical phase of recovery. We discuss the nutritional elements crucial for supporting muscle repair and overall well-being in Parkinson's patients, ensuring that the recovery process aligns seamlessly with their health objectives.

Exercise Modalities for Parkinson's Patients

- ***Tailoring Exercise Programs:*** Recognizing the diversity of physical capabilities in Parkinson's patients, we explore the integration of tailored exercise modalities, encompassing aerobic, strength, and flexibility training to address individual needs and challenges.

Parkinson's Diet for Enhanced Performance

- ***Nutritional Support for Optimal Performance:*** The discourse extends to nutritional approaches that amplify exercise performance. We identify specific foods and supplements beneficial for stamina, recovery, and sustained physical activity in Parkinson's management.

Common Challenges and Solutions

- Addressing Unique Hurdles: Acknowledging prevalent challenges such as swallowing difficulties during exercise, we propose adaptive solutions. Additionally, we explore ways to adjust diet plans to support and complement varying levels of physical activity.

Holistic Wellness: Mental Health and Exercise

- Psychological Benefits: Shifting focus to holistic wellness, we examine the positive impact of exercise on mental health and cognitive function.

Nutritional interventions that support mental well-being in conjunction with physical activity are scrutinized.

Creating a Personalized Diet and Exercise Plan

- ***Collaborative Approach:*** Highlighting the significance of collaboration between individuals with Parkinson's, their healthcare professionals, and nutritionists, we underscore the creation of personalized diet and exercise plans. This section encourages ongoing feedback and adjustments to optimize individualized strategies over time.

Real-life Success Stories

- ***Inspirational Narratives:*** The discourse concludes with inspirational narratives, exemplifying individuals who have thrived through the symbiotic integration of diet and exercise. Practical tips and lessons learned from these stories offer a beacon of hope and guidance.

Tailoring Nutrition to Support Physical Activity

The synergy between nutrition and physical activity forms the cornerstone of overall health and well-being. This professional discourse delves into the intricacies of tailoring nutrition to support physical activity, particularly in the context of individuals grappling with Parkinson's disease. In understanding the specific needs of this population, we embark on a journey to explore the symbiotic relationship between diet and exercise for optimal health outcomes.

Understanding the Unique Needs of Parkinson's Patients

- ***Disease-Specific Considerations:*** Parkinson's disease introduces distinct challenges that influence both nutritional requirements and the body's response to physical activity. Recognizing these nuances is crucial in developing a tailored approach to support individuals on their journey towards a more active and healthier lifestyle.

Pre-Exercise Nutrition Strategies

- ***Nutrient Timing and Composition:*** Before engaging in physical activity, the body requires a strategic infusion of nutrients. This section explores the importance of pre-exercise nutrition, detailing optimal nutrient timing and composition to enhance energy levels, support endurance, and facilitate a more effective exercise session.

Hydration and Electrolyte Balance

- ***Essential Components for Exercise:*** Hydration emerges as a fundamental pillar in supporting physical activity. We dissect the critical role of water and electrolytes in maintaining fluid balance, preventing dehydration, and sustaining individuals throughout their exercise routines.

Post-Exercise Nutritional Considerations

- ***Facilitating Recovery:*** The post-exercise phase is a critical period for recovery and muscle repair. We delve into the nutritional considerations essential for Parkinson's patients after physical activity, emphasizing the significance of a well-rounded approach to optimize recovery and overall well-being.

Addressing Swallowing Difficulties During Exercise

- ***Practical Solutions:*** Swallowing difficulties are not uncommon in Parkinson's patients and can pose challenges during physical activity. This section provides practical solutions and adaptive strategies to overcome these hurdles, ensuring that individuals can comfortably and safely engage in exercise.

Adapting Diet Plans to Varying Levels of Physical Activity

- ***Flexibility in Nutrition:*** Acknowledging the diversity in physical capabilities among individuals with Parkinson's, we explore the importance of flexibility in diet plans. Tailoring nutritional strategies to accommodate varying levels of physical activity is emphasized, promoting sustainability and individualized support.

Personalized Nutrition Counseling

- ***Collaborative Approaches:*** Highlighting the importance of a multidisciplinary approach, we discuss the role of personalized nutrition counseling. Collaboration between individuals with Parkinson's, healthcare professionals, and nutritionists is pivotal in crafting tailored nutrition plans that align with specific health goals and address unique challenges.

Realizing the Cognitive Benefits of Nutrition

- ***Mental Well-being and Cognitive Function:*** Beyond the physical aspects, we explore the cognitive benefits of nutrition in supporting mental well-being and cognitive function. Nutritional interventions that contribute to enhanced cognitive performance are discussed within the context of promoting a holistic approach to health.

Building a Holistic Approach to Health

In the pursuit of well-being, a holistic approach to health stands as an integral paradigm that transcends mere physical considerations. This professional discourse aims to illuminate the multifaceted nature of holistic health, particularly within the context of individuals navigating the complexities of Parkinson's disease. By weaving together physical, mental, and nutritional facets, we endeavor to construct a comprehensive framework that fosters resilience, vitality, and an enhanced quality of life.

Embracing the Multidimensional Nature of Health

- ***Beyond the Physical:*** Holistic health transcends the physical realm, recognizing the intricate interplay between mental, emotional, and nutritional components. Understanding and addressing each dimension is fundamental in constructing a robust foundation for overall well-being.

Mental Well-being in Parkinson's

- ***The Mind-Body Connection:*** Exploring the profound impact of mental well-being on physical health, particularly in the context of Parkinson's disease, unveils the intricate mind-body connection. Strategies to promote emotional resilience and cognitive health are integral elements of a holistic health approach.

Nurturing Physical Resilience

- ***Integrating Exercise into Daily Life:*** Physical activity is not merely a component of health; it is a catalyst for resilience. Tailoring exercise regimens to the unique needs of Parkinson's patients and integrating movement seamlessly into daily life constitute essential facets of fostering physical well-being.

Nutrition as a Pillar of Health

- ***Customizing Dietary Approaches:*** The significance of nutrition extends beyond sustenance, playing a pivotal role in supporting health. Tailoring dietary approaches to meet the specific needs of individuals with Parkinson's fosters not only physical nourishment but also contributes to comprehensive health.

The Power of Lifestyle Modifications

- ***Beyond Medication:*** Lifestyle modifications, encompassing exercise routines, dietary adjustments, and mindfulness practices, emerge as powerful allies in Parkinson's management. These modifications complement medical interventions, contributing to a holistic strategy for optimal health.

Integrating Holistic Practices

- ***Collaborative Healthcare:*** A holistic approach involves collaboration between healthcare professionals, including neurologists, nutritionists, and mental health practitioners. This collaborative effort ensures that individuals with Parkinson's receive comprehensive care that addresses the diverse facets of their well-being.

Empowering Individuals

- ***Education and Self-Care:*** Empowering individuals with knowledge about holistic health principles and self-care practices is a cornerstone of this discourse. By fostering a sense of agency and understanding, individuals can actively contribute to their overall health and engage in informed decision-making.

Realizing Holistic Success Stories

- ***Inspirational Narratives:*** To illuminate the effectiveness of a holistic approach, this discourse culminates in real-life success stories. These narratives showcase individuals thriving with Parkinson's, embodying the transformative power of a comprehensive, multidimensional health strategy.

CHAPTER THIRTHEEN

EMOTIONAL WELL-BEING AND NUTRITION

Addressing Emotional Eating

In the complex tapestry of eating behaviors, emotional eating emerges as a significant aspect that intertwines food and emotions. This discourse delves into the nuanced phenomenon of emotional eating, particularly within the context of Parkinson's disease. By exploring the psychological underpinnings, identifying triggers, and fostering healthy coping mechanisms, we aim to guide individuals towards cultivating a balanced and mindful relationship with food.

Understanding Emotional Eating

- ***Unraveling the Connection:*** Emotional eating involves the consumption of food in response to emotions rather than hunger. In the realm of Parkinson's, understanding the intricate relationship between emotions and eating behaviors becomes paramount for cultivating a holistic approach to health.

Recognizing Triggers

- ***Uncovering Emotional Catalysts:*** Identifying triggers that prompt emotional eating is a pivotal step. This section explores common triggers within the context of Parkinson's and provides insights into recognizing the emotional undercurrents that drive such behaviors.

Coping Mechanisms Beyond Food

- ***Healthy Alternatives:*** In the journey towards mitigating emotional eating, exploring alternative coping mechanisms is imperative. Strategies for managing stress, anxiety, and other emotional states without resorting to food become integral components of fostering emotional well-being.

Mindful Eating Practices

- ***Cultivating Awareness:*** Mindful eating emerges as a powerful tool to counteract emotional eating tendencies. This section delves into practices that encourage present-moment awareness, fostering a mindful approach to food consumption within the Parkinson's community.

Tailoring Nutrition to Emotional Well-being

- ***Nourishing the Mind and Body:*** Examining the role of nutrition in emotional well-being provides insights into dietary choices that support mental health. The interplay between certain nutrients and mood regulation is explored, offering a holistic perspective on nourishing both the mind and body.

Seeking Professional Support

- ***Collaborative Approaches:*** Addressing emotional eating often requires a collaborative effort. In this section, the discourse highlights the importance of seeking professional support, including mental health professionals, nutritionists, and Parkinson's care specialists, to guide individuals towards a healthier relationship with food.

Personal Narratives and Success Stories

- ***Inspirational Journeys:*** To inspire and resonate with readers, this discourse concludes with personal narratives and success stories. These stories highlight individuals within the Parkinson's community who have successfully navigated and overcome emotional eating, providing hope and practical insights for others on a similar journey.

Mindful Eating Practices

In a world marked by fast-paced lifestyles and constant distractions, the concept of mindful eating emerges as a transformative approach to nourishing both the body and mind. This discourse delves into the essence of mindful eating practices, offering insights and practical guidance for individuals, particularly those navigating the challenges of Parkinson's disease. By fostering a mindful approach to food, individuals can cultivate a deeper connection with their eating experiences and promote overall well-being.

Understanding Mindful Eating

- ***The Essence of Presence:*** Mindful eating involves being fully present during meals, engaging all the senses to savor and appreciate the eating experience. Within the context of Parkinson's, this practice takes on added significance in promoting a holistic approach to health.

Embracing the Senses

- ***Savoring the Culinary Experience:*** This section explores the importance of engaging the senses-taste, smell, sight, touch, and hearing-during meals. Embracing the sensory richness of food enhances the overall eating experience and fosters a deeper connection with nutritional choices.

Cultivating Awareness of Hunger and Fullness

- ***Tuning into Body Signals:*** Mindful eating encourages individuals to attune to their body's signals of hunger and fullness. Recognizing and respecting these signals forms a foundational aspect of mindful eating practices, contributing to a healthier relationship with food.

Breaking Free from Distractions

- ***Unplugging During Meals:*** The discourse emphasizes the detrimental effects of distractions, such as screens and external stimuli, during meals. Practical tips for creating a conducive environment for mindful eating, even in the midst of a busy world, are explored.

Practicing Gratitude and Reflection

- ***Nourishing the Mind and Soul:*** Incorporating gratitude practices and moments of reflection during meals enrich the emotional and mental aspects of eating. This section explores techniques for fostering a positive and appreciative mindset around food.

Mindful Eating for Digestive Health

- ***Enhancing Nutrient Absorption:*** Mindful eating contributes to improved digestion by promoting a relaxed state during meals. Understanding the connection between mindful practices and digestive health within the Parkinson's context is discussed.

Tailoring Mindful Eating to Parkinson's Challenges

- ***Adapting Practices for Unique Needs:*** Addressing the challenges posed by Parkinson's, this section provides insights into tailoring mindful eating practices to accommodate motor difficulties, swallowing issues, and other specific concerns.

Integrating Mindful Practices into Daily Life

- ***Sustainable Lifestyle Shifts:*** The discourse concludes by exploring strategies for seamlessly integrating mindful eating practices into daily life. Emphasizing that mindfulness is a skill that can be cultivated over time, the discourse encourages individuals to embark on this transformative journey towards greater awareness.

Seeking Support for a Positive Relationship with Food

Cultivating a positive relationship with food is a journey that often benefits from external support and guidance. In the context of Parkinson's disease, where unique challenges may arise, seeking appropriate support becomes even more crucial. This guide explores various avenues and strategies individuals can explore to foster a positive and nourishing relationship with food, enhancing overall well-being.

Professional Guidance

- ***Nutritionists and Dietitians:*** Engaging with nutrition experts, such as registered dietitians or nutritionists with experience in Parkinson's care, provides tailored advice. These professionals can help individuals create personalized dietary plans that align with their health goals, considering both physical and emotional aspects.

- ***Mental Health Professionals:*** Collaborating with psychologists, counselors, or therapists specializing in eating behaviors can be instrumental. These professionals can offer support in addressing emotional aspects tied to food and developing coping mechanisms for a healthier relationship with eating.

Support Groups

- ***Parkinson's-specific Support Groups:*** Participating in Parkinson's support groups creates a community where individuals can share experiences, challenges, and successes related to their relationship with food. Peer support fosters a sense of understanding and camaraderie, reducing feelings of isolation.

- ***Online Communities:*** Virtual platforms provide accessible spaces for connecting with others facing similar challenges. Online forums, social media groups, or dedicated websites centered around Parkinson's and nutrition offer valuable insights and support.

Family and Friends

- ***Building a Supportive Network:*** Educating close family and friends about the challenges and goals related to food and Parkinson's can create a supportive environment. Having a network that understands and encourages positive habits contributes significantly to well-being.

Mindfulness Practices

- ***Incorporating Mindful Eating Techniques:*** Integrating mindfulness practices, such as meditation and mindful eating exercises, can be empowering. Learning to be present during meals, recognizing hunger and fullness cues, and appreciating the sensory aspects of food are skills that support positive eating habits.

- ***Yoga and Relaxation Techniques:*** Engaging in activities like yoga or relaxation exercises contributes to an overall sense of well-being. These practices can help manage stress, which is often linked to emotional eating, and promote a positive mindset towards food.

Parkinson's Organizations and Resources

- ***Utilizing Educational Materials:*** Organizations dedicated to Parkinson's often provide educational materials and resources. These materials may include guidelines, meal plans, and tips tailored to individuals with Parkinson's, empowering them to make informed choices.

- ***Educational Events and Webinars:*** Attending events or webinars hosted by Parkinson's organizations can provide valuable insights. Experts often share advice on nutrition, lifestyle, and coping strategies, fostering a proactive approach to managing the relationship with food.

Holistic Wellness Programs

- ***Comprehensive Well-being Initiatives:*** Exploring holistic wellness programs that encompass nutrition, exercise, and mental health can be beneficial. These programs are designed to address multiple facets of well-being and offer a structured approach to fostering a positive relationship with food.

CONCLUSION

In conclusion, a well-managed and carefully curated diet can play a crucial role in supporting individuals with Parkinson's disease. While there is no one-size-fits-all approach, emerging research suggests that certain dietary patterns and nutritional components may positively impact Parkinson's symptoms and overall well-being.

A diet rich in antioxidants, vitamins, and minerals, particularly those found in fruits, vegetables, and whole grains, appears beneficial for individuals with Parkinson's disease. These nutrients may help mitigate oxidative stress and inflammation, which are implicated in the progression of the disease. Additionally, maintaining an adequate intake of protein while balancing it with other macronutrients is essential, as protein absorption can be affected in Parkinson's patients due to medication interactions.

Furthermore, some studies suggest that specific diets, such as the Mediterranean or anti-inflammatory diet, may offer neuroprotective effects and contribute to better outcomes for Parkinson's patients. These diets emphasize the consumption of fish, olive oil, nuts, and a variety of colorful fruits and vegetables, all of which contain compounds with potential anti-inflammatory and neuroprotective properties.

However, it is crucial for individuals with Parkinson's disease to work closely with healthcare professionals, including dietitians and neurologists, to tailor dietary recommendations to their specific needs and medication regimens. Factors such as medication interactions, individual nutritional requirements, and any existing medical conditions must be considered when developing a personalized dietary plan.

In conclusion, while diet alone cannot cure Parkinson's disease, it can be a valuable and complementary aspect of a comprehensive approach to managing the condition. Combined with appropriate medical treatment, regular exercise, and a supportive lifestyle, a well-balanced and nutritionally sound diet can contribute to improved quality of life for individuals living with Parkinson's. Continued research in this field will likely provide further insights and refine dietary recommendations for better symptom management and overall well-being.